COPING V

FIONA MARSHALL has written widely on health, psychology and parenting. She is the author of several Sheldon Press books, including *Living with Autism* and *Your Man's Health*, and also a novel.

Overcoming Common Problems Series

Selected titles
A full list of titles is available from Sheldon Press,
1 Marylebone Road, London NW1 4DU, and on our website at
www.sheldonpress.co.uk

Assertiveness: Step by Step
Dr Windy Dryden and Daniel Constantinou

Body Language at Work
Mary Hartley

The Cancer Guide for Men
Helen Beare and Neil Priddy

The Candida Diet Book
Karen Brody

The Chronic Fatigue Healing Diet
Christine Craggs-Hinton

Cider Vinegar
Margaret Hills

Comfort for Depression
Janet Horwood

Confidence Works
Gladeana McMahon

Coping Successfully with Hay Fever
Dr Robert Youngson

Coping Successfully with Pain
Neville Shone

Coping Successfully with Panic Attacks
Shirley Trickett

Coping Successfully with Prostate Cancer
Dr Tom Smith

Coping Successfully with Prostate Problems
Rosy Reynolds

Coping Successfully with RSI
Maggie Black and Penny Gray

Coping Successfully with Your Hiatus Hernia
Dr Tom Smith

Coping with Alopecia
Dr Nigel Hunt and Dr Sue McHale

Coping with Anxiety and Depression
Shirley Trickett

Coping with Blushing
Dr Robert Edelmann

Coping with Bronchitis and Emphysema
Dr Tom Smith

Coping with Candida
Shirley Trickett

Coping with Childhood Asthma
Jill Eckersley

Coping with Chronic Fatigue
Trudie Chalder

Coping with Coeliac Disease
Karen Brody

Coping with Cystitis
Caroline Clayton

Coping with Depression and Elation
Dr Patrick McKeon

Coping with Down's Syndrome
Fiona Marshall

Coping with Dyspraxia
Jill Eckersley

Coping with Eczema
Dr Robert Youngson

Coping with Endometriosis
Jo Mears

Coping with Epilepsy
Fiona Marshall and
Dr Pamela Crawford

Coping with Fibroids
Mary-Claire Mason

Coping with Gallstones
Dr Joan Gomez

Coping with Gout
Christine Craggs-Hinton

Coping with a Hernia
Dr David Delvin

Coping with Incontinence
Dr Joan Gomez

Coping with Long-Term Illness
Barbara Baker

Coping with the Menopause
Janet Horwood

Coping with a Mid-life Crisis
Derek Milne

Coping with Polycystic Ovary Syndrome
Christine Craggs-Hinton

Coping with Psoriasis
Professor Ronald Marks

Overcoming Common Problems Series

Coping with SAD
Fiona Marshall and Peter Cheevers

Coping with Snoring and Sleep Apnoea
Jill Eckersley

Coping with Stomach Ulcers
Dr Tom Smith

Coping with Strokes
Dr Tom Smith

Coping with Suicide
Maggie Helen

Coping with Teenagers
Sarah Lawson

Coping with Thyroid Problems
Dr Joan Gomez

Curing Arthritis – The Drug-Free Way
Margaret Hills

Curing Arthritis – More Ways to a Drug-Free Life
Margaret Hills

Curing Arthritis Diet Book
Margaret Hills

Curing Arthritis Exercise Book
Margaret Hills and Janet Horwood

Cystic Fibrosis – A Family Affair
Jane Chumbley

Depression at Work
Vicky Maud

Depressive Illness
Dr Tim Cantopher

Effortless Exercise
Dr Caroline Shreeve

Fertility
Julie Reid

The Fibromyalgia Healing Diet
Christine Craggs-Hinton

Getting a Good Night's Sleep
Fiona Johnston

The Good Stress Guide
Mary Hartley

Heal the Hurt: How to Forgive and Move On
Dr Ann Macaskill

Heart Attacks – Prevent and Survive
Dr Tom Smith

Helping Children Cope with Attention Deficit Disorder
Dr Patricia Gilbert

Helping Children Cope with Bullying
Sarah Lawson

Helping Children Cope with Change and Loss
Rosemary Wells

Helping Children Cope with Divorce
Rosemary Wells

Helping Children Cope with Grief
Rosemary Wells

Helping Children Cope with Stammering
Jackie Turnbull and Trudy Stewart

Helping Children Get the Most from School
Sarah Lawson

How to Accept Yourself
Dr Windy Dryden

How to Be Your Own Best Friend
Dr Paul Hauck

How to Cope with Anaemia
Dr Joan Gomez

How to Cope with Bulimia
Dr Joan Gomez

How to Cope with Stress
Dr Peter Tyrer

How to Enjoy Your Retirement
Vicky Maud

How to Improve Your Confidence
Dr Kenneth Hambly

How to Keep Your Cholesterol in Check
Dr Robert Povey

How to Lose Weight Without Dieting
Mark Barker

How to Make Yourself Miserable
Dr Windy Dryden

How to Pass Your Driving Test
Donald Ridland

How to Stand up for Yourself
Dr Paul Hauck

How to Stick to a Diet
Deborah Steinberg and Dr Windy Dryden

How to Stop Worrying
Dr Frank Tallis

The How to Study Book
Alan Brown

How to Succeed as a Single Parent
Carole Baldock

How to Untangle Your Emotional Knots
Dr Windy Dryden and Jack Gordon

Hysterectomy
Suzie Hayman

Overcoming Common Problems Series

Overcoming Common Problems

Coping with Down's Syndrome

Fiona Marshall

sheldon **PRESS**

First published in Great Britain in 2004 by
Sheldon Press
1 Marylebone Road
London NW1 4DU

Copyright © Fiona Marshall 2004

British Library Cataloguing-in-Publication Data

A catalogue record for this book is available from the British Library

ISBN 0–85969–921–8

1 3 5 7 9 10 8 6 4 2

Typeset by Deltatype Limited, Birkenhead, Merseyside
Printed in Great Britain by Biddles Ltd
www.biddles.co.uk

Contents

To all families
with a child who has
Down's syndrome

Acknowledgements

The Down's Syndrome Association; the National Society for
Epilepsy for information on Down's syndrome and epilepsy; and all
those who so generously shared their experience of bringing up a
child with Down's syndrome, including Annabel Tall, of London,
mother of Freddie, Jo Dawson, of London, mother of Luke, and
Miriam Kauk, of Southwestern Indiana, mother of Mary, for her
useful leads and tips, and Victor Bishop and the Bishop family in
Southwestern Illinois, for striking historical facts.

Introduction

'I look forward to the day when a mongolian idiot, treated biochemically, becomes a successful geneticist.' This quote is from the French doctor Jérôme Lejeune, deploring the practice of aborting babies with Down's syndrome. His words go to the heart of many issues surrounding those with Down's syndrome, in particular, their dignity within society.

Perceptions of Down's syndrome are changing. Just 100 years ago, babies with Down's syndrome were routinely institutionalized. Some 50 years ago, parents might still have been encouraged to have an 'afflicted' baby 'put away'. Some readers of this book may be among those who remember shameful playground taunts of 'Mongol, Mongol!' to an unpopular child. Even ten years ago, the future for a child with Down's syndrome was not as bright as it is today.

In the past few years, much has changed. It is not merely that 'mongolism' is out (as outdated as 'idiot', used as a medical term in Victorian times), institutions are definitely out or that old-fashioned shame and dismay around Down's syndrome are going out. Today, there is a growing realization of the potential for children with Down's syndrome – so much so that at times it seems like an entirely different condition to that described just a few years ago.

For a start, modern medicine can do so much more for children with Down's syndrome that their quality of life, as well as life expectation, is vastly improved. Much suffering is avoided. While, sadly, some children do go through wretched periods of ill health and may remain fragile, many families are also free to develop the potential of their children at a much earlier age than was possible previously.

There is greater emphasis on early intervention – working with children at an early age to develop their capabilities – and on inclusion, ensuring that children attend mainstream school and keep up with their peers right into secondary school and beyond. Motor, cognitive and social development are all areas of breakthrough for children with Down's syndrome. We are still discovering how much they can do and all that they can be.

Above all, there is growing acceptance of children with Down's syndrome as children. Children with a variety of temperaments, interests and abilities, children who play, squabble with siblings, do schoolwork, swim, misbehave, go on holiday, attend groups, clubs and so on. The birth of a baby with Down's syndrome is, first and foremost, a new baby to welcome, a new life to celebrate.

Ignorance and negativity do still exist. The doctor who breaks the news with bleak warnings about the child's likely future, the relative full of patronizing myths such as 'At least he'll always be loving and good', the friend who arrives at the new mother's bedside with eyes full of tears and sympathy.

In the age of the designer baby, in a competitive, results-orientated culture, a child with Down's syndrome is still an embarrassment to some, hard to colonize in contemporary society. However, any baby is an embarrassment to a former lifestyle, any baby upsets expectations, changes values, stretches ideas of love, sometimes to the limit, maybe tramples over career prospects and personal comfort. The reality of any baby (as opposed to the fantasy baby that may be carried during a pregnancy) can be lovely, lonely, difficult. It's just that a baby with Down's syndrome presents a reality for which new parents are even less prepared than the reality of a new baby without Down's syndrome.

When you first learn that your baby has Down's syndrome, you may feel overwhelmed by a variety of emotions. Shock, anger, fear and acute loneliness are natural. You may have outdated ideas of what Down's syndrome is floating round in your mind, you may wonder how you are going to cope or how others will react; almost certainly there will be a period of grieving for the baby you did not have. It's a time of special vulnerability for new parents. Even if you were prepared for your baby by antenatal tests, there will still be a period of readjustment.

Information and sharing with other parents can be paths through this difficult period – when you are ready. It may take days, weeks or months before you feel able to start taking in the facts. In time, however, finding out about Down's syndrome and learning how other families have managed can be extremely helpful, lessening feelings of isolation and giving hope in an unfamiliar, new life where all the landmarks have to be learned afresh.

It is hoped that this book, which sets out to present an updated view of Down's syndrome, will help to give you that information. There are many other excellent resources for families with a child who has Down's syndrome and these are given at the end of the book in the Further reading and Useful addresses sections. This book is a starting point, but it is also very worthwhile contacting the Down's Syndrome Association – a most helpful organization with comprehensive literature and access to different sources of support.

The work and ethos of such organizations are part of a modern approach to Down's syndrome, representing an ideal that is becoming reality against the social odds. In the words of the world-famous expert on Down's syndrome, Dr Siegfried Pueschel, 'When accorded their rights and treated with dignity, people with Down's syndrome will, in turn, provide society with a most valuable humanizing influence.'

Editor's note

In the UK, the terminology 'Down's syndrome' is generally used, so this is what we have used in the book. However, in the names of some organizations, medical texts and the USA, it is 'Down syndrome', so this form is used when referring to such organizations and so on.

1

Welcoming your baby

'Your baby has Down's syndrome.' If, like most parents, you have heard these words just after the birth of your child, you are probably experiencing a range of emotions, the like of which you never anticipated. After nine months of expectation, you've given birth to this vulnerable, mysterious being whom you haven't yet had time to get to know. Now others have stepped in and branded your baby with a title that makes him or her a double stranger. Maybe even before you've decided on a name, the medical profession has given him or her a label of its own. Shock, disbelief, anger and other elements of grief are natural reactions.

What is Down's syndrome and how exactly does it affect the child? Is it life-threatening? How can new parents cope with an apparently formidable range of special needs as well as the ordinary demands of parenthood, which seem overwhelming enough? These and many more questions may be coursing through your head even as you hold or change the small person who is responsible for them.

Hearing the news

It was my first baby and I was still very dazed from delivery – I'd been in labour for 30 hours and had had forceps. I couldn't really take in what the midwife was talking about when she said she wanted to fetch a colleague to take a look at the baby; of course she already knew. There was a hush in the delivery room. The midwife came back with the registrar. He was young and matter of fact and slightly distant, but told me as kindly as possible that my baby had Down's syndrome. It was awful. The midwife started crying – she told me later she'd been off sick for several months and this was her first delivery back at work. They then took the baby off for lots of tests and I didn't see her again for four hours. I thought she was going to die.
Tiffany, mother of Jacquie, 5

The hospital was incredibly good. A very kind doctor and a senior sister broke the news to us. They arranged for us to come into a private room with the baby and told us that Tara looked healthy and bouncing but that they had unexpected news for us; she had Down's syndrome. They asked us if we had any questions, but we were too shocked, we just sat there in silence. So then they told us a lot more about Down's syndrome and how the prospects for such children had improved vastly these days, how they could learn to do practically all the things other children do, if more slowly – talk, walk, play and learn. Nothing can ease the shock of hearing this kind of news about your baby, but the way they told us did make for the best possible start. They also put us in touch with another couple who'd had a baby with Down's syndrome several months previously and this was a great help.
Sean and Moira, parents of Tara, 2

The staff were obviously trying to be kind but you couldn't help feeling that they regarded the baby as a mistake rather than a human being and couldn't wait to get rid of us. The two doctors who told us came across as condescending and abrupt respectively. The abrupt one insisted on telling us as much as possible about the health problems related to Down's syndrome and kept saying, 'You might as well know.' His favourite phrase seemed to be 'early mortality'. He told us that it was unlikely the child would amount to much as a social being and we'd better change our entire expectations about parenthood (later we did but probably not in the way he meant!). The condescending one talked about how there was no reason why Down's syndrome children shouldn't live a full life, but in a way that seemed to cut them off from the rest of the human race. Once they'd said their piece they both got up and walked out with no time for us to ask questions. We were left feeling incredibly alone and very frightened, as if we'd been abandoned with a being from outer space, not a baby.
Ruth, mother of Jack, 3

Unfortunately, the news about the baby is usually heard soon after delivery, which is an especially vulnerable time, when the mother may be exhausted after labour and some 40 weeks of pregnancy, or dazed by the reality of the small, new being who has arrived and now needs care 24 hours a day. Some women feel vulnerable in a hospital setting, too. There may be acute anxiety over a baby who is poorly. As they struggle to adapt to the facts about their baby, new mothers may also have to cope with the baby blues two or three days after the birth, when the very high levels of pregnancy hormones drop and other hormones involved in milk production arrive, causing weepiness and irritability. All in all, most women are not in the best shape at such a time to hear this kind of news.

Down's syndrome is one of the few conditions featuring intellectual disability that parents learn about before they have had a chance to bond with their baby. Most other conditions (such as autism) become apparent only when the baby is a toddler or older and often as a dawning realization on the part of parents rather than a sudden shock.

It is well recognized that how the news is broken has a massive impact; few parents ever forget it. It is equally accepted that some ways of breaking the news are better than others. Research shows that most parents want to know as soon as possible, together and with the baby there.

Obviously, a positive, gentle approach is appreciated, with time for parents to ask as many questions as they want. Unfortunately, some health professionals still have an outdated approach to Down's syndrome or may feel that it is their duty to warn parents of possible problems ahead (not usually thought necessary with any other baby who may actually be just as much trouble or more). However, there is increasing emphasis on education for health professionals as to the best, most dignified way of breaking the news.

Some parents find out that their baby has Down's syndrome during the pregnancy. This is a whole separate issue and so is covered in Chapter 5, Diagnosis – antenatal tests.

Your reactions

Freddie was born with a rare condition in which his intestines had formed on the outside of his body. He was so sick that we didn't get to grips with the Down's syndrome aspect for about a month, and then we were just so glad that he was alive.
Annabel

You can only see one day at a time – the shock element is so great. After Luke was born, we were put in touch with a lovely couple who had a little girl of nine months with Down's syndrome. They told us that time would make it better and we just couldn't understand this. Now when I meet new mums, their pain is palpable and I can relate to it so well.

I don't know how I turned that corner, but one day I was able to take Luke out without that burden of worry that everyone would be looking at me with pity or wondering how I could have gone ahead and had this child. You can't rush the process – some people may not take as long as I did, others may take far longer.
Jo

It will take time to adjust to this new reality – perhaps months, perhaps years. Your whole expectations of parenthood have to be reappraised on a deep level. Many parents go through a grieving process. This grief may be for the child you dreamed of having, but who will never be; for your own future as parents; for the opportunities and achievements you fear your child will now miss; for many lost dreams and expectations. Grief covers a range of emotions, including denial and anger, eventually mingling with growing acceptance. Once over the initial shock, though, many parents come to acceptance in time; new challenges bring new rewards, and parents learn to delight in their child – personality and achievements – but the early days with the expected or unexpected news about your baby often bring a flood of turbulent feelings.

Not all parents go through the following emotions, but they are common as you come to grips with the reality of your newborn baby.

- *Shock* Shock may be felt physically – you may feel sick, faint or cold. Inability to take in information is a feature of shock, so although you may have just spent half an hour with the doctor, you might not be able to remember much of what he or she said or you might feel that no one has told you anything or that new medical terminology is being used that you just don't understand. Alternatively, you may just feel blank or unable to connect.
- *Denial* You may feel that the doctors must have made a mistake or simply that it can't happen to you and your family. Some parents may even have an anxiety that their own baby has been secretly or inadvertently exchanged with another baby (the changeling myth).
- *Fear* Many parents are terrified at the news that they have received. There may be fear of the unknown, fear that the child will be severely affected, fear of rejection by society, fear of how family and friends will react. There may be siblings to consider or

worry about how your partner will react. Fear of the future can be particularly harrowing – how will you manage once alone at home, never mind in years to come? Will the baby die? What about milestones such as starting school, learning or making friends? Most of these fears turn out to be unfounded, but seem very real and bleak at the time.

- *Anger* It is natural to feel extremely angry that this has happened to you. Anger is deeply bound up with feelings of loss. Rage may be general or may be expressed as anger towards medical carers, your partner, with grandparents or with other family members or friends.

- *Guilt* You may be afraid that you have caused your child's condition, despite assurance from doctors that this is impossible. Guilt here may involve anything from having had an alcoholic drink in pregnancy to fear that this is divine punishment for some misdemeanour or a feeling that you have inherited a faulty family gene. Some parents worry that their child has met with an accident while no one was looking – that the baby was dropped by a nurse, for example, or didn't get enough oxygen in the first few minutes after birth. This is all part of the thinking that your child's condition could and might have been prevented and is a profound aspect of grief. It takes time to come to terms with this kind of powerless remorse.

- *Feelings towards your child* It is important to realize that these may be ambivalent with any newborn baby. Speak to anyone who has experienced post-natal depression and you will soon see that the rosy image of the fulfilled new mother is not the whole story. A new baby means new responsibilities, less freedom and a complete change of identity, which some people find very threatening. For some, it takes time and support in order to adapt. Sadly, many new mothers today just don't get enough support, but are expected to battle on entirely on their own. Feeling ambivalent or negative towards your baby is natural – it doesn't mean that feelings of love don't coexist with these other feelings, too.

Post-natal depression

Post-natal depression is different from the baby blues and may kick in weeks or even months after the birth. One of the main feelings is that of not being able to cope. You may also feel angry, irritable, weepy, negative towards your baby, very depressed, even suicidal.

Changes in your usual eating and sleeping patterns may also occur.

There is debate over the cause. Some experts believe that it is a hormonal problem, while others feel it is due to a combination of factors following a profound life change, including social isolation, stopping work and taking on the huge responsibility of a new baby.

Do see your doctor as soon as possible, who should be able to suggest some treatment, such as putting you in touch with a local post-natal support group (often made up of other mothers) counselling and psychotherapy, medication and alternative therapies (aromatherapy, reflexology and others).

It is also worth contacting the National Childbirth Trust or the Association for Post Natal Illness for information and advice (see the Useful addresses section at the back of the book).

Adoption

Occasionally, some parents feel that they cannot cope with the fact that their baby has Down's syndrome and may need to talk about the possibility of fostering or adoption with a hospital social worker. Most parents prefer to keep their babies once they have got to know them, but a small number do proceed with adoption or foster care. Some couples wishing to adopt specifically request a baby with Down's syndrome, feeling that they have a special contribution to make in this area. It is also not unknown for parents to have decided on adoption and then changed their minds shortly afterwards. One couple got home, thought better of it and rushed back to hospital to retrieve their baby, luckily before any paperwork had been made out. Normally, changing your mind is not an option.

As you readjust

New mothers need time to rest after the very hard work of childbirth. Whether you're in hospital or at home, try to get enough rest – this will help you to recover quickly, and also to cope with your early emotions. Ask your partner to limit visitors if need be, especially if you feel that you have to keep explaining about the baby over and over again. Just see people you know you can trust.

It's well accepted that a new mother needs mothering herself. Do accept any 'maternal' offers of help, whether it's housework, nappy-changing or – perhaps most important – just being there for you. Don't try to do it all alone unless you really have to.

This is also a time when new mothers need the best possible nutrition. Again, accept all offers of help and make sure that you eat well. Drinking enough fluid is also important, especially if you are breastfeeding – at least eight glasses of water a day.

Above all, do make time to welcome and enjoy your baby. As Ruth says, 'I'd really advise new parents just to enjoy those baby moments. They pass so fast. We were so consumed by anxiety that I think we missed a lot of Jack just being a baby.'

Telling others about your new baby

As soon as you feel able, it can be extremely helpful just to let people know about your new baby. Many parents feel very isolated by what has happened and telling others does help break through these feelings. The news of a new baby should be spread and celebrated.

Be prepared for the news to be met with a range of reactions – from simple lack of understanding to warm acceptance. Bear in mind that others will probably follow your lead, so, the more positive you can be in presenting the news, the better.

While friends may try to be supportive, not all of them may be able to accept the reality of a baby with Down's syndrome, either. Others, though, will prove sterling. Many parents find strong support from new friends met via support groups.

> Friends are key. Some are unable to get involved – one such even asked us, 'Are you going to get it adopted?' – but other friends are so inclusive there's no divide. I don't know what I would have done without friends.
> *Jo*

For those who do react negatively, sadly, it's their loss. You will probably find that most people rally to your side, ready to support you and share in your experiences with your baby. Indeed, your experience may well cause you and others to reflect and revalue what is important in life.

As we have seen, even in the medical profession, knowledge of Down's syndrome tends to be limited and outdated. For example, it may not always be realized that children with Down's syndrome today have a far wider range of educational and community opportunities than children born even a decade ago. Likewise, health prospects and life expectancy are both vastly improved. So, you may need to educate others, but maybe not just yet! For now, a general statement is probably enough – perhaps to the effect that things have changed so much with regard to what is known about Down's syndrome.

Grandparents, like parents, can grieve over the loss of the 'normal' grandchild they expected to have. In addition, grandparents are concerned about the stress and difficulties they may anticipate for their children.

> My mother-in-law has been fantastically supportive – Tara could have been her own baby. My own mother has had great difficulty accepting Tara. She'll still say things like, 'I've been to Lourdes praying for a cure,' when she knows full well there is no cure for Down's syndrome.
> *Moira*

In time, most grandparents come to accept and love their special grandchild profoundly.

Talking to others about your feelings

Once the news has been broken, you may find that you now want to talk to someone about your conflicting emotions. For some, this may mean reappraising former friends before you settle on someone with whom you feel at ease. Again, this tends to happen after the birth of any baby – you may find that you have less in common with work colleagues and can talk to other new mothers more easily, for example.

Finding other parents of children with Down's syndrome can be an immense source of strength and support (see the Useful addresses section at the back of the book for contact details if your hospital doesn't put you in touch with a local group).

This wonderful couple came in with their baby, Jasmine, who was 11 months old. They told us that we'd take time to readjust, but that we would adjust and that there was a lot of help available – early intervention programmes. We would see our baby progress and develop. And we would love her to bits. It all came true.
Sean and Moira

Some people may find it easier to clam up as they may feel stronger alone or feel that they don't want to burden their partner, friends or relatives. There may indeed be a time when silence is your best friend, when it hurts too much to talk. If you can't or don't want to talk in these early days, respect this and don't feel obliged to share feelings when you are not ready.

Some people also find it a challenge to be open and honest with their partners. They may feel the need to keep a brave face in front of the other person or be supportive of him or her at a difficult juncture in their lives. Some couples do benefit from a neutral time when deep discussion gives way to getting to grips with the practicalities of life with a new baby, but, at some point, pooling your strength through open discussion is a lot more effective than keeping emotions to yourself.

A baby first and foremost

To sum up, try not to make or listen to any negative predictions at this time. Down's syndrome spans a wide range of abilities and health conditions and no one can know in advance what your child will accomplish in life – which is true of all children. Your baby is a baby first and foremost. He or she will be totally dependent on you for everything, just as all other babies depend on their parents. Like all other babies, too, he or she will eat, sleep a great deal and go through lots of nappies. He or she may have some medical problems, but will also be very much in need of your love and very ready to love you back. Your baby's needs are identical to the needs of all other babies. As Annabel says, 'I have three wonderful sons, one of whom just happens to have Down's syndrome.'

2

About Down's syndrome

Down's syndrome is the most common of all genetic conditions and it would appear to have been with us for quite some time. According to the world-famous authority on Down's syndrome, Dr Siegfried Pueschel, a Saxon skull from the seventh century shows alterations in its structure that only appear in children with Down's syndrome, while aspects of the syndrome are believed to appear in ancient works of art, suggesting that, in the past, these children had a special place in various societies.

Today, Down's syndrome affects 1 in every 800 to 1000 babies – that's approximately 3000 to 5000 births per year in the United States, while 2 babies with Down's syndrome are born every day in the UK. These figures are much lower than the actual conception rate, but many Down's syndrome babies are lost naturally at some time during pregnancy, while other parents decide on termination (see Chapter 5, Diagnosis – antenatal tests). There are some 60,000 people in the UK with Down's syndrome and more than 350,000 people in the United States.

So, what is Down's syndrome? Unlike many gene defects, which happen because a key gene is missing, in most cases of Down's syndrome, the baby is formed with three, rather than the usual two, copies of chromosome 21, so giving the child 47 instead of 46 chromosomes, and with an extra copy of certain genes on the third chromosome 21. This means that they are producing too much of certain body chemicals, throwing into disarray the finely tuned mechanisms that govern the development and functioning of vital organs.

The effects of Down's syndrome vary widely, with very differing degrees of intellectual impairment. As yet, however, it is impossible to predict how severely a baby will be affected. Some people believe that there is a 'window of opportunity' in babyhood, during which time brain damage may be prevented by taking the right supplements. This is a controversial issue, however, and by no means medically proven (more on this in the section on diet in Chapter 9). What is certain is that your input from an early age will help your child achieve his or her maximum potential. Today, there is a great deal of emphasis on early intervention and there are many ways in which you can contribute to your child's cognitive, motor and overall development. Some ideas for things to try are explored later in this book.

As well as resulting in learning disability, Down's syndrome also carries an increased likelihood of various health problems. Sadly, some babies are born very sick indeed and may need a period of intensive hospital care before being able to go home. Others may be mildly affected by two or three conditions, while yet others may have just one persistent problem that will need to be treated by means of routine medical care. However, many children with Down's syndrome today are robust and healthy.

Some health conditions are more serious than others – particularly congenital heart disease. Your baby is also likely to be more prone to infections, especially of the respiratory kind, so you may need to keep an eye open for early signs of any sinus and chest infections. Some children will also have vision and hearing problems or other medical conditions, such as an obstructed digestive tract.

Daunting as this sounds when rolled off as a list like this, thanks to modern medicine, these conditions are treatable. The health of people with Down's syndrome has been vastly improved by the availability of antibiotics and advances in heart surgery. For more on health, see Chapter 6, Health issues.

What distinguishes children with Down's syndrome?

John Langdon Haydon Down, who identified Down's syndrome, was struck by the physical similarities between those who had Down's syndrome – so much so that he commented on an overall family or racial likeness these children seemed to share. (Down's original well-meaning 'racial' theory has been thoroughly discredited and, indeed, he himself discarded much of it during his lifetime – see Chapter 3.) Today there is much more emphasis on the fact that children with Down's syndrome are individuals who resemble their families far more than they do each other – especially now that we no longer see them in the drab, uniform garments that were doled out by Victorian institutions, which is how Down would have seen them, but, like other children, sporting the whole variety of modern children's clothes. Most parents today will look for family resemblances in their baby – that he has his uncle's expression or looks like his siblings when they were babies, though he will probably have some of the facial traits associated with Down syndrome as well.

A 'syndrome' is a group of characteristics, and there are more than 100 different characteristics associated with Down's syndrome. No single child with Down's syndrome will have every one of these characteristics. Some will have quite a lot and others will have only a few. Like all children, those with Down's syndrome are hugely different from each other in terms of appearance, abilities and personalities, as well as attitudes and interests.

Typical physical features, however, include the following.

- Floppiness owing to reduced muscle tone (hypotonia). This often improves as your baby gets older.
- Distinctive almond-shaped eyes with an upward and outward slant, often with a fold of skin running vertically between the two lids at the inner corner of the eye (the epicanthic fold).
- Flattening of the back of the head, with a low hairline and often rather loose skin at the nape of the neck.
- A small nose with a flattened nasal bridge and rather flat facial features.
- A small mouth with a slightly protruding, large-looking tongue. In fact, true enlargement of the tongue (macroglossia) is rare – more often, the tongue is a normal size, but the mouth is smaller because of underdevelopment of the mid-face.
- Fairly broad hands with short fingers – the little finger curving inwards.
- A single crease across the palm of the hand (palmar or simian crease). Palmar creases develop early in pregnancy, by the time the unborn baby is 11 to 12 weeks old. While abnormalities in palmar creases are associated with developmental disorders such as Down's syndrome, a single palmar crease, or simian crease, is found to occur naturally in approximately 1 out of 30 people. Males are twice as likely as females to have this type of crease.
- Hyperflexibility – the baby is more flexible or 'bendy' than usual because the ligaments, which hold joints together, are slacker. For example, you might notice that your baby's legs lie flatter than usual when you are changing him or her.
- A space between the first and second toes – sandal gap.
- Shorter than usual height. In babies, you will see a below average weight and length at birth.

Other typical features include distinctive grey or very light yellow spots on the iris of the eyes (Brushfield's spots) and small, low-set ears. These are the sorts of features that will be looked for by a medical professional who is diagnosing Down's syndrome, but otherwise they have no real significance – that is, they cause no significant disability in the child. In addition, many of these features can be found in people who do not have Down's syndrome. For example, 4 to 5 per cent of children who do *not* have Down's syndrome have a single crease across their palm, 6 to 8 per cent of children without Down's syndrome display epicanthic folds and 25 to 50 per cent of people who do not have Down's syndrome have slanted eyes, flat back of the head, small ears and flat nasal bridge.

Down's syndrome dolls

The special characteristics of a baby with Down's syndrome are celebrated in an exceptional way by an American company that has created dolls faithfully reflecting the appearance of a baby with the condition.

The dolls – Down Syndrome Originals© – are the dreamchild of Donna Moore of Downi Creations in Irmo, South Carolina – a non-profit organization working to raise awareness of Down's syndrome.

While working with children with disabilities, Donna Moore felt that, as children with Down's syndrome are drawn to others with the same condition, she felt that such children would enjoy and benefit from having a doll that was like them.

The dolls, created by designer Jerri McCloud, reflect the 'special beauty' of babies with Down's syndrome by faithfully representing the 13 features of the syndrome, including slanted eyes, a flat bridge across the nose, a small mouth with a visible tongue, small ears, small hands with short fingers and a single crease in the palm of each hand. The little fingers curve inwards and each foot has a gap between the first and second toe of the flat feet. Also, reflecting the fact that many of these children have heart defects that need surgery, a red heart with stitches is embroidered on the doll's chest. (See the Useful addresses section at the back of the book for contact details.)

Other features of Down's syndrome

While the extra genetic material will affect your child's physical and mental development, it is no longer expected to confine his or her potential. With vastly improved health prospects and life expectancy, support from professionals and groups and a more modern outlook on the syndrome, there is every prospect of a full life ahead. It is generally expected that children with Down's syndrome will reach the same developmental milestones as other children, if at a slower rate, but this varies.

One area of delay is mental development. Down's syndrome results in varying degrees of learning difficulty, from mild to severe. Speech and language development is also slower. Physical development will be slower, too, and your child will probably be later than is typical in achieving milestones such as rolling over, sitting and crawling. For example, while the average age for walking is 12 to 14 months, children with Down's syndrome may learn to walk around 15 to 36 months. However, as mentioned above, love and stimulus from you will go a long way towards helping your child's development, as will intervention and help from others. Indeed, it is not really possible to predict future development. Many children with Down's syndrome today have progressed well beyond expectations.

Researchers have investigated the idea of a Down's syndrome 'personality' for more than a century, but inconclusively. Certain studies have looked at whether or not those with Down's syndrome are 'easier' and 'happier' than other people. A study at the Western Isles Hospital, Isle of Lewis, Scotland, found that those with Down's syndrome were less likely to demonstrate maladaptive behaviour than were people with other disabilities. Another study, by Leila Ricci and Robert Hodapp of the University of California, Los Angeles, looked at fathers of children with Down's syndrome versus other types of intellectual disability. It found that both fathers and mothers rated their children with Down's syndrome as having more positive personality traits and less maladaptive behaviour, while fathers also reported less child-related stress.

Many parents have given testimony to the creativity, tolerance and feistiness of their special children. Down himself noted their sense of humour and social intelligence: 'They have considerable power of imitation, even bordering on being mimics. They are humorous and a lively sense of the ridiculous often colours their mimicry.'

As regards the popular sentimental idea of the Down's syndrome child – happy, affectionate and musical – this is another matter. Most parents contacted for this book greeted the idea with hoots of derision, followed by a carefully qualified description of an individual child who was sometimes content and sometimes cross and who enjoyed a wide range of activities that might or might not include music. In their personalities – as in their appearance, intellectual ability and development – children with Down's syndrome remain individuals.

Tests and checks that your baby may have

Even if it seems fairly certain that your baby has Down's syndrome, a chromosome test needs to be done before making a final diagnosis. A tiny sample of blood is taken from the baby and the chromosomes analysed. The result is called a *karyotype* and shows the three copies of chromosome 21 in 94 per cent of cases. (The other 6 per cent have other chromosomal abnormalities, as described in Chapter 4, Causes and types of Down's syndrome.)

There are various other tests your baby may have if he or she is believed to have Down's syndrome.

- A physical examination will pick up any of the obvious physical signs described above, as well as other typical indications of Down's syndrome. A doctor may also listen for a heart murmur by listening to the baby's chest with a stethoscope.
- X-rays may be taken to see whether or not your baby has any heart abnormalities or intestinal blockages.
- Your baby may have an echocardiogram, to see if there are any heart problems. This is a test that uses sound waves to create a moving picture of the heart. The picture is much more detailed than an X-ray image and involves no radiation exposure.
- An electrocardiogram (ECG) records the electrical activity of the heart. It is used to measure the rate and regularity of heartbeats, as well as the sizes and positions of the chambers and the presence of any damage to the heart.

Your baby may well cry during tests, but don't worry – this is a normal response to the strange environment and people, restraints and separation from you rather than them hurting in any way. You yourself may become anxious about the procedures being carried out. Ask your doctor if it is possible for you to stay with your baby during the tests, especially if the procedure allows you to maintain physical contact as this will reassure you both.

Can Down's syndrome be treated medically?

Although many medications and various therapies have been suggested as treatments for those with Down's syndrome, it is not a disease and there is no effective medical treatment as such at the present time. However, there is much that can be done to improve a child's quality of life and minimize developmental delays. Also, of course, any related health conditions are treatable. In fact, parents have found that it is important to ensure that these *are* treated and not mistaken as being part of the syndrome. For example, constant crying and refusal to eat or sleep could be due to an ear infection. Poor feeding and floppiness are characteristic of Down's syndrome, but may also be indicative of heart disease (early checks should indicate whether or not your baby has any heart conditions). It is always worth checking out worrying symptoms or behaviour with your doctor to rule out routine or more severe illness.

Treatments and therapies to improve Down's syndrome itself have been touted. One 'treatment' is cell therapy, popular in Germany. This involves injecting the person with Down's syndrome with cells from newborn or foetal animals. A study of cell therapy by Dr Stanley Levin of the Schneider Children's Hospital, New York, concludes that it is worse than useless and, further, carries dangers of causing potentially fatal allergic reactions, infections and, later, autoimmune disease. The money, concludes Dr Levin, would be better spent at accredited child development centres to forward a child's progress. Sometimes extravagant claims have also been made for nutritional programmes. Again, this needs a balanced approach. Obviously, your child will benefit from a healthy diet, but the issue of supplementation is covered in more detail in Chapter 9.

What of the future?

In 1959, Dr Jérôme Lejeune discovered the genetic cause of Down's syndrome (see Chapter 3) and hoped to find a treatment therapy. He argued that if we could understand the effect these extra genes had on the development and growth of the child, it should be possible to develop a treatment therapy to cancel out that effect. For the moment, however, treatment has yet to catch up with Lejeune's ground-breaking work. Genetic therapy – whether by altering the gene itself or developing medicines to impact on the gene's effects – remains a possibility for the future. Chapter 4 looks at some of the research in progress in this field.

3

Some history

Medical recognition of Down's syndrome is comparatively new, but the syndrome itself is believed to have existed from antiquity. For example, it has been speculated that ancient Olmec statues bear a striking resemblance to the facial features of Down's syndrome. These figures were made by the Olmecs, who lived along the Gulf Coast in what is now southern Mexico between 1500 and 300 BC. Of course it may equally be the case that the statues record certain facial features typical of the Olmecs, but the slanting eyes and epicanthic folds are distinctive.

It has also been suggested by Andy Merriman in his book *A Minor Adjustment*, about his daughter Sarah who has Down's syndrome, that certain Renaissance artists, such as Andrea Mantegna, painted angels and babies with the characteristics of Down's syndrome children – perhaps as symbols of enduring innocence. Suggestive features include the positioning of the ears – further back than is usual – and the gap between the big and other toes. The angels surrounding the Madonna della Humilità, painted in about 1437 by the Carmelite friar Filippo, may also be viewed as having certain characteristics of Down's syndrome.

A Saxon skull from the seventh century, noted by Dr Siegfried Pueschel, the authority on Down's syndrome, may be the oldest anthropological find relating to Down's syndrome. The skull shows typical features in its structure that only appear in those with the syndrome.

What is certain is that Down's syndrome was an integral part of human diversity long before it was officially recognized by medical practitioners.

Before Down

In 1866, when John Langdon Haydon Down first described the syndrome that bears his name, he mentioned his surprise that it had not been described earlier. He was wrong, however. In fact, features of the syndrome were described in 1838 by Jean Etienne Dominique Esquirol (1772–1840), a founder of modern alienism (the study of mental diseases). Esquirol is known for *Des Maladies Mentales considérées sous les Rapports Médical, Hygiénique et Médico-Légal,* which he published in Paris in 1838. Called 'the first complete psychiatrist', Esquirol founded a mental institution where he lived among his patients, and he was ahead of his time in believing that an individual approach needed to be taken with each one.

Another clinical description was made by Edouard Séguin (1812–80) in 1844. Séguin revolutionized methods of teaching children with serious mental handicaps. With Jean Marie Gaspard Itard (1774–1838), he was the inspiration for Maria Montessori – founder of the world-famous system of education. Itard was a doctor who worked with the deaf and mentally challenged, for whom he evolved an educational system. He was famed for his discovery of Victor the Wild Boy of Aveyron in France in 1799.

John Langdon Haydon Down

In 1866, John Langdon Haydon Down made the first detailed description of the syndrome that bears his name. Down himself – an unusual and charismatic person whose place in medical history has only recently been recognized – is the fascinating subject of a book by Irish doctor O. Conor Ward, former professor of paediatrics, University College Dublin.

Down was indeed a 'caring pioneer', as O. Conor Ward put it in the title of his book, *John Langdon Down: A Caring Pioneer* (unfortunately out of print). An early advocate for training those with mental disabilities, Down started an institution for mentally disabled children, Normansfield, which was the first of its kind and gained an international reputation. Here, according to their ability, patients were taught life skills such as self-care, cooking, how to handle money and buying and selling, along with hobbies such as dancing, gymnastics, music, languages and sports. Activity was also provided in the form of entertainments, outings and caring for the institution's 40 acres of farmland, which included a well-known herd of black and white pigs. By treating patients as human beings with a full range of potential, Down revolutionized the care of those with mental disabilities.

In addition to his work on Down's syndrome, Down also described Prader-Willi syndrome, which is a chromosomal disorder characterized by obesity.

He was forward-thinking and liberal in other ways, too, lending out his Harley Street consulting rooms to suffragettes as part of his support for women's liberation. He strongly disagreed with the popular belief that higher education for women would make them likely to give birth to 'feeble-minded' babies!

Down's advice to his medical students was to aim high. He added that the secret of success in life was 'earnest and persistent work', supplemented by a 'gentle Christian life.'

Down, who left school at 14, was inspired to undertake a medical career by a kind of visionary compassion after meeting what was then called a 'feeble-minded' girl. 'The question haunted me – could nothing for her be done? . . . the remembrance of that hapless girl presented itself to me and I longed to do something for her kind.'

After a rather grim medical apprenticeship in the East End, where he learned such skills as blood-letting and tooth extraction, Down qualified as a pharmacist at 18. He then entered medical school at the London Hospital, where he proved a brilliant student and won medals and awards.

Expected to have a brilliant career at the university hospital, he caused surprise when, in 1858 – a time when mentally disabled children were gravely neglected – he became superintendent of the large Royal Earlswood Asylum for Idiots in Surrey, sharing his time between there and his London practice.

After making numerous reforms, Down turned Earlswood into a renowned facility, a model of its kind. It was here that Down began classifying patients.

He died a wealthy, renowned and much-loved man in 1896. Shops were shut for his funeral and members of the public stood on the pavement in silent tribute as his cortège passed by. A street was named in his honour in Teddington and another in Torpoint. 'Surprisingly his life story has not attracted the attention it deserves,' comments O. Conor Ward.

How Down classified children

Down based his findings on head skull shapes and palate sizes. In this he was much influenced by ethnology, which traced a relationship between the shape of the skull and how far developed the brain was beneath. Anthropology was also fashionable at the time and the classification of head shapes in different races was thought to correlate with different potential learning skills (see 'Down and racism' below).

To make his diagnoses, Down also used several clinical photographs – a field in which he was also a pioneer. Indeed, his collection of some 200 photographs is the largest known archive of Victorian clinical photography.

Down noticed that certain children shared the same type of appearance. Indeed, the similarities were so striking that they appeared to all come from the same family. Down speculated that these children were a 'throwback' to another race – the ancient Mongolian race, hence the term 'mongolism' or 'Mongolian idiocy'.

Down's first paper on the subject, 'Observations on an ethnic classification of idiots' (1866), stated that:

> The boy's aspect is such, that is difficult to realize that he is the child of Europeans . . . The face is flat and broad and destitute of prominence. The cheeks are roundish and extended laterally . . . The tongue is long, thick and much roughened. The nose is small. The skin has a slight dirty yellowish texture and is deficient in elasticity, giving the impression of being too large for the body.

Down speculated that all this was the result of 'degeneration' stemming from tuberculosis in the parents. He went on to observe that many of the children had poor coordination, their circulation was feeble and they showed delayed development during the winter, suggesting that some of them had thyroid problems.

Down also noted that this group of patients responded very well to training, doing better than would be expected. Their life expectancy, however, was below average and they tended to develop tuberculosis.

In 1876, Down identified the fold of skin at the inner corner of the eyes – the epicanthic fold – and the position of the ears, which is usually further back than in other children. Down's son Reginald described the single crease across the palm of the hand in 1908, though it is not clear whether this was his own discovery or he was reporting what he had learned from his father. Reginald Down himself had a son with Down's syndrome in 1905. Although Reginald's wife Jane found this hard to accept, the boy became a well-loved member of the family, living to the ripe old age of 65.

The characteristic grey or yellowish spots on the iris of the eye were noted by the English doctor Thomas Brushfield (1858–1937) in 1924 and so have since been known as Brushfield's spots.

Down and racism

Down has been criticized for being racist, but, like many other great men, he was a product of his time. It was an era when the language of scientific naturalism was increasingly used to explain the behaviour of the dangerous classes in Victorian society, such as criminals, or to explore uncomfortable issues, such as the place of women, racial differences, poverty, insanity and alcoholism. The medical community generated much of this discussion.

In Down's day, it was widely believed that five distinct races existed in the world: Mongolians, Aztecs, Caucasians, Malayans and Ethiopians. Europeans considered that the 'Caucasian race' was superior to the 'Mongoloid race' in intellect. Down tried to classify all the Earlswood residents according to one or other of these racial groups.

Down's ethnic classification never came to be widely accepted and, indeed, he himself abandoned it in due course. All that is now remembered of it is his description of what he described as the 'Mongolian type', a description that evolved into what we now term Down's syndrome. Strange as it seems to modern sensibilities, the terms 'idiot' and 'imbecile' were also used as accepted medical terms at the time.

'Mongolism' and 'Mongoloid' persisted into the 1960s and 1970s, but, in 1961, a group of genetic experts wrote to the *Lancet* suggesting that the condition be renamed. Down's syndrome was the term chosen, and this was confirmed by the World Health Organization in 1965. In the 1970s, an American revision of scientific terms changed it simply to 'Down syndrome', although it still is most usually called 'Down's syndrome' in the UK.

Prejudice and ignorance

Down's original observation on the children in his care was that, 'They are cases which very much repay judicious treatment.' Alas, his words were sadly ignored for over 100 years.

As recorded by Victor Bishop, who runs the Riverbend Down Syndrome Parent Support Group, in 1946 Benjamin Spock – the major child-rearing authority at the time, whose book, *Baby and Child Care*, was a parents' bible – suggested that babies born 'mongoloid' should at once be placed in an institution on the grounds that they were 'hardly human'.

In 1968, theologian Joseph Fletcher, trying to comfort a bereaved parent, said 'a Down's is not a person.' As late as 1970, the *Encyclopaedia Britannica* listed for the last time Down's syndrome under the heading 'Monster'. For other historical facts, visit Victor Bishop's Down's syndrome timeline at: www.altonweb.com/cs/downsyndrome/timeline.html.

Michel Foucault (1926–84) described in his book *Madness and Civilization* (1984) how, in the seventeenth century, the asylum (in other words, prison or confinement) was intended to deal with poverty and economic crises throughout Europe. This spatial seclusion was not just a place, but a whole social, administrative structure to deal with those perceived to be a threat to society. He wrote: 'The community acquired an ethical power of segregation, which permitted it to eject, as into another world, all forms of social uselessness.'

Thankfully, a more modern outlook is prevailing with the work of doctors such as Jérôme Lejeune, who provided another turning point in the history of Down's syndrome.

Jérôme Lejeune (1929–94)

Jérôme Lejeune and colleagues discovered the chromosomal nature of Down's syndrome in 1959 in France, and this has proved to be the foundation for modern research. Patricia Jacobs and colleagues also discovered the forty-seventh chromosome in England almost simultaneously.

Known as the father of modern genetics, Lejeune discovered numerous illnesses that have genetic origins and was an ardent defender of life and of the dignity of 'those who are mentally wounded', as he called them.

Contrary to the popular view that the tiny baby becomes more and more developed as the weeks of pregnancy go on, Lejeune posited that the very first cell, the fertilized egg, is 'the most specialized cell under the sun'. Lejeune firmly believed that life begins at conception when 'the whole necessary and sufficient genetic information is gathered inside one cell, the fertilized egg'. This fertilized egg, according to Lejeune, contains more information about the being than can be stored in five sets (not volumes, sets) of the *Encyclopaedia Britannica* (if enlarged to normal print size).

> At no time is the human being a blob of protoplasm. As far as your nature is concerned, I see no difference between the early person that you were at conception and the late person which you are now. You were, and are, a human being.

Lejeune was vitally interested in treating those with Down's syndrome as living beings, and his research into the biochemistry of Down's syndrome that he started continues today. He recognized the importance of folic acid in optimizing intelligence in these children. He also realized that the 'floppiness' characteristic of many was due to thyroid dysfunction. He investigated the usefulness of various amino acids in treating this condition, along with the antioxidant vitamins A, C and E (see Chapter 9 for details of current research into these topics).

The work of the Lejeune Foundation in Paris continues to research the causes and mechanisms of Down's syndrome, as well as develop possible therapies. It funds and conducts a wide range of studies that vary from, for example, infantile spasms in babies with Down's syndrome to how the medicine folinic acid may help prevent further mental disability in children with Down's syndrome.

The Down's Clinic in London also continues Lejeune's research. Originally called the Lejeune Clinic, it opened in the Hospital of St John and St Elizabeth in 1995 and has been so successful that a further clinic has been opened in Liverpool and there are plans for others in the West Country and the Midlands. The clinic in London is run by a team of paediatricians, psychologists, haematologists and speech therapists and treats children from all over the UK. The medical team has investigated several issues in children with the syndrome and found that many of them have iron deficiency and some have congenital high blood cholesterol levels. These problems can be treated easily and doing so helps to improve their intelligence.

While the clinic does have a waiting list (treatment is complementary to ongoing medical care), there is no reason not to give your child a diet that is rich in iron and folic acid – both of which have been isolated by researchers at the Down's Clinic as being important for children with Down's syndrome. Foods rich in iron include beef, oysters, sardines, poultry, cod, wheatgerm, lentils, soya beans, molasses, baked potato skins, cocoa powder, quinoa, seaweed, dried apricots and curry powder. Folic acid is found in fortified cereals and bread, oranges, dark green leafy vegetables, dried peas and beans, nuts and seeds (use as a paste rather than whole for small children, unless they have allergies and then avoid altogether). See Chapter 9 for more information about diet.

4

Causes and types of Down's syndrome

The exact cause of Down's syndrome is unknown. It appears to be an accident of nature and, in the vast majority of cases, is not hereditary. It is certain that it is a genetic event, one that is more likely to take place in older mothers, but, beyond that, no reason for the condition has been established. This may be deeply frustrating and saddening for those who like to know just why and how their baby was affected. There is an understandable need to find meaning in cause and effect. Indeed, gaining this understanding can be an important part of the grieving process.

One question that may cause parents particular anguish is whether or not they did anything to cause the syndrome in their baby or if it could have been prevented. Rest assured that the answer to both of these questions is no. Down's syndrome occurs at the moment of conception or before and there is no known parental behaviour that impacts on it.

Looking for causes can be an emotionally charged issue, as there may be a temptation to blame yourself, others or events for the outcome. Tiffany, mother of Jacquie, said it was a relief to realize that her actions and behaviour during pregnancy had had no effect on her baby.

> I'd been over every little incident during pregnancy wondering if I'd eaten the wrong thing – perhaps it was that alcoholic drink I'd indulged in before I knew I was pregnant – but no. It was reassuring to realize that the syndrome occurs even before the baby has formed that first cluster of cells, and so my actual pregnancy had nothing to do with it. Even after I knew that, rationally, it took me a long time to accept it emotionally. I felt very guilty and responsible, and felt other people were looking at me and blaming me, as if I'd had some kind of choice in the matter.
> *Tiffany*

Blaming yourself is an understandable part of the process of coming to terms with what has happened. However, it does not really stand up to logical examination. Blaming yourself is essentially an emotional or moral response to a stochastic process ('stochastic' means involving a random variable, chance or probability). To put it in perspective, it is an accepted fact that approximately 1 to 1.5 per cent of all new babies will have some sort of abnormality. Apportioning blame for this is not appropriate.

There are many theories as to what could cause Down's syndrome, including hormonal abnormalities, the effect of X-rays, viral infections and problems with the immune system. Stress during pregnancy has been suggested, but this can be dismissed due to the certain knowledge that Down's syndrome occurs at or before conception.

Folic acid and Down's

Some research has suggested that taking folic acid before pregnancy might reduce the chance of having a baby with Down's syndrome. It is a well-established good practice to take extra folic acid before conception and during pregnancy as it has been shown to protect against neural tube defects, such as spina bifida (when the neural tube, which becomes the brain and spinal cord, develops abnormally in early pregnancy).

One study has found that families with a high incidence of neural tube defects also have an unexpectedly high incidence of Down's syndrome. Researchers led by Howard Cuckle, Professor of Reproductive Epidemiology at the University of Leeds, studied around 1000 families and speculated that abnormal metabolism of folic acid might underlie both neural tube defects and Down's syndrome.

Folic acid is available as a supplement, but foods rich in folic acid include orange juice, poultry, liver; leafy green vegetables such as spinach, broccoli, borlotti, haricot and kidney beans, lentils, fortified breakfast cereals, enriched grain foods such as bread, rolls, rice and pasta, and enriched flours.

It is important that parents of children with Down's syndrome understand that these findings should not be a source of guilt or anxiety – parents should not blame their child's condition on their own diet before and during pregnancy. A single study is not conclusive. You should also consult your doctor about your individual needs for folic acid before deciding to supplement.

How Down's syndrome occurs

Down's syndrome occurs in three ways, although one of them is by far the most common, accounting for 95 per cent of all cases. This is *non-disjunction* or *trisomy 21* ('trisomy' means triplication, referring to the three copies of chromosome 21). Occasionally there is only an additional *part* of chromosome 21, and this is known as *partial trisomy 21*.

The two other types of chromosomal abnormalities are rarely involved in Down's syndrome, but do occur. They are known as *mosaicism* and *translocation*.

Non-disjunction or trisomy 21

Non-disjunction is when certain cells fail to divide properly, resulting in an embryo with three number 21 chromosomes instead of two. What happens is that a pair of number 21 chromosomes in either the sperm or the egg fail to separate. As the embryo develops, the extra chromosome is replicated in every cell of the body. Of course, if conception never takes place, the presence of the fault is of no reproductive significance.

The fact remains that this cause of Down's syndrome – or what we know about it – often begins even before conception. Because this is so, and we know that the faulty cell division often exists in the woman's egg before conception and that women are born with their complete lifetime store of eggs, it has been speculated that some environmental factors may be implicated in non-disjunction. However, despite years of research, the cause of non-disjunction is still unknown, the only proven factor being older motherhood.

Translocation

As with non-disjunction or trisomy 21, translocation occurs either before or at conception and is found in 3 to 4 per cent of those with Down's syndrome. Unlike non-disjunction, there is no link between the age of the mother and the chance of translocation. Most cases appear to be random, accidental events in which the extra chromosome 21 moves across (hence, it is translocated) to attach itself to another chromosome – usually chromosome 14, 21 or 22.

However, in around a third of cases, there is a genetic factor and one parent – either the father or the mother – may be a carrier of a translocated chromosome. For this reason, the chance of recurrence for translocation is higher than that of non-disjunction. Genetic counselling can be sought to determine the origin of the translocation.

Mosaicism

Mosaicism – which occurs in around 1 per cent of cases of Down's syndrome – is when two types of cells become mixed with some of the cells containing 46 chromosomes and some containing 47. Those cells with 47 chromosomes contain an extra chromosome 21. This error is believed to take place shortly after conception. The term mosaicism is used because of the 'mosaic' pattern of the cells.

Some research suggests that babies with mosaic Down's syndrome may be less affected than those with trisomy 21. However, as has already been mentioned, people with Down's syndrome do have a wide range of abilities so it is hard to generalize.

Older mothers

It is well known that the chance of having a baby with Down's syndrome increases with the age of the mother, but why are older mothers more vulnerable to having an affected baby?

'Older mothers' are so-called as a hangover from the days when women would start having babies in their teens. Age-related chance is based on the simple fact that every woman is born with all of her eggs (oocytes) and they age along with her chromosomes and the rest of her body. In effect, this means that the ovum, or egg, that forms one part of the developing baby at conception is as old as she is. So, for example, if you are 35, you have 35-year-old eggs and if you are 35 and your mother was 25 when she conceived you, then you are the product of an egg that developed 60 years ago! So, given that many body functions decline with age, it may be that the eggs of an 'older mother' may simply be past their prime.

Another theory is that the eggs may have been exposed, over a woman's lifetime, to external environmental factors, such as radiation, or internal ones, such as medication. Another suggestion by Dr Janet Carr, author of *Down's Syndrome: Children Growing Up* (1995), is that all women have a certain number of eggs containing the extra chromosome. As a woman only has a set number of eggs, the affected ones will be used last by the body.

There are other theories, too, as to why older mothers are more likely to have babies with Down's syndrome than younger mothers.

One is that the woman is nearing the end of her reproductive life so that the body does its best to hang on to what may be its last pregnancy and ensure it goes to term, even if the baby is affected by a chromosomal abnormality. At least 50 per cent of early (first trimester – that is, first three months) miscarriages are pregnancies with a major chromosomal abnormality. The rate of trisomic conceptions (babies with Down's syndrome) are the same at all ages, but such pregnancies are more likely to go to term in older women rather than end in miscarriage. This theory is linked to a phenomenon known as the ovary's 'last fling' – a surge of fertility sometimes experienced by women aged in their late thirties or early forties, resulting in a little surprise addition to the family. A body where fertility is declining tends to hang on tightly to any chance to conceive and bear a child.

What are the chances of having a Down's syndrome baby?

The chances of having a Down's syndrome baby have always been assessed by maternal age – the older the mother, the greater her chances of having a baby with the condition. However, a child with Down's syndrome can be born to a mother at any age.

The chances are calculated approximately as follows, according to figures from the Wolfson Institute, St Bartholomews Hospital, London.

Age of mother	Chances of having a baby with Down's syndrome
25	1 in 1351
30	1 in 909
35	1 in 384
38	1 in 189
40	1 in 112
45	1 in 28
50	1 in 6

However, while statistically the chances are greater for older mothers, in fact more babies with Down's syndrome are born to younger women – 80 per cent of children with Down's syndrome are born to women who are less than 35 years old (51 per cent to mothers under 30, and 72 per cent to women under 35). Although only 5 to 8 per cent of pregnancies occur in women over the age of 35, they account for 20 per cent of Down's syndrome births.

Because of higher fertility rates in younger women, this group makes up the largest number of mothers and screening for Down's is routinely offered only to older mothers.

Chances of having further children with Down's syndrome

What about the chances of having another child with Down's syndrome? In fact, this happens more rarely than statistics would suggest. In theory anyway, the chances of a parent of a child with trisomy 21 having another child with Down's syndrome is approximately 1 in 100. If, however, your child's Down's syndrome was due to translocation, genetic counselling and chromosome analysis is advised as the chances of this recurring may be much greater, depending on the type of translocation and whether the translocation is carried by the father or the mother.

Older fathers

Until recently, it was believed that the mother was the sole source of the extra genetic material that causes Down's syndrome. However, there has been interest in the father as a possible contributor to the condition.

Some research suggests that men in midlife or older may share their mature partner's increased genetic mutational liability – in other words, that older fathers may also have an increased chance of being the source of the extra chromosome 21. Some studies have suggested that older fathers are responsible for 25 per cent of Down's syndrome. This genetic liability has been well-established with other genetic disorders. One large study showed that there is an increased rate of schizophrenia in adult children of older fathers (those who become fathers in their late forties to sixties). Such a connection is well-established with other conditions, too, such as the rare achondroplasia (dwarfism).

31

Fathers, like mothers, are getting older. Data from the Office for National Statistics (ONS) reveals that, in 1971, the average age of a father at the birth of their child was 27 years, but, by 1999, this had risen to 30.

What happens is that, as men become older, their sperm reproduces by means of division. Each successive division introduces a slight chance of error in the genetic material of the new sperm, which is then passed on to the child.

About chromosome 21

When Jérôme Lejeune discovered the genetic cause of Down's syndrome, a cure seemed to be ruled out on the grounds that genetic inheritance cannot be changed. However, Lejeune still hoped to find a therapy. His focus was on targeting the metabolic consequences of having the extra genes. He posited that, if we could understand the effects that these extra genes had on the development and growth of the child, it should be possible to develop a therapy to cancel out these effects. However, as the extra set of genes is identical to the other two sets at chromosome 21, this raises the question of how one set might be turned off without affecting the other two sets.

Since then, Down's syndrome has commonly been viewed as irreversible. However, in the last 10 to15 years, much more has been discovered about the brain, thanks largely to much more sophisticated brain-scanning techniques. Some scientists believe that the brain's plasticity theoretically leaves it open to treatment for Down's syndrome, but research into this (some of which is outlined below) is in its early stages and any treatment is still some way off.

Scientists in Germany and Japan have managed to decode chromosome 21 – the focus of much scientific interest due to its association with Down's syndrome, among other factors. Identifying the complete code of chromosome 21 brings the possibility of genetic therapy a little nearer. By understanding the chromosome, scientists believe that it will be easier to identify Down's syndrome and other diseases and any individual causes due to the workings of individual genetic material.

These researchers are also looking at how the extra genetic material throws out of balance the rest of a person's genetic make-up, so leaving him or her more vulnerable to other genetic and environmental insults, leading to the features, diseases and conditions associated with Down's syndrome.

The body's 23 chromosomes contain approximately 30,000 genes. Given that there are identical copies of each chromosome, that's a total of 60,000 per person. The extra genes associated with Down's syndrome are believed to form a mere handful – some estimates put it at maybe around 20. Chromosome 21 itself has around 225 genes. Genetically, then, people with Down's syndrome are heavily weighted towards 'normality'. The extra genes are also in themselves 'normal' genes. It remains for scientists to discover just why and how a few extra genes impact on development so as to cause Down's syndrome.

Genetic research into Down's syndrome

A long-term series of studies is aiming to take genetic research a few stages further towards actual treatments. By analysing the cognitive development of those with Down's syndrome, scientists hope to provide tools for treatment – whether it is more refined intervention and education or even corrective gene 'mapping' – that is, tinkering with the gene itself so as to minimize the effects of Down's syndrome. These therapies may also be used in treating other forms of mental disability and diseases such as Alzheimer's disease.

To take just one example, scientists at the Universities of Denver, Colorado and Arizona have studied the brains of those with Down's syndrome. The scan images suggest that they are different from the brains of those who do not have Down's syndrome. Areas studied include the prefrontal cortex, which controls functions such as paying attention, controlling impulses, planning and organization; the hippocampus, associated with long-term memory; and the cerebellum, in charge of motor functions, such as balance and coordination, and also implicated with learning and attention. For example, a link has been found between problems with learning and memory and a loss of cholinergic neurons (those parts of the brain that use acetylcholine as a neurotransmitter – acetylcholine is vital for mental functions such as memory and planning and also causes muscle fibres to contract).

The scientists are looking at ways in which the learning styles of children with Down's syndrome may differ from those of children with other developmental disorders. For example, they may be strong in areas such as social knowledge, but have greater problems in others, such as memory. Children with Down's syndrome may also vary greatly from one another in their abilities. By analysing the functioning of the brain in greater detail and linking their discoveries to genetic knowledge, scientists hope to design treatments that are as closely modelled as possible to the genetic realities of chromosome 21.

Other scientists are conducting research that could one day lead to drugs being developed that reverse some of the symptoms of Down's syndrome. For example, scientists at Stanford University Medical Center, California, and the University of Geneva are focusing on understanding the biological cause of the condition, down to the specific genes responsible for the varied symptoms. For example, a gene known as COL6A1 may be responsible for heart defects, while superoxide dismutase (SOD1) may cause premature ageing and weakening of the immune system. Once these have been definitively identified, the researchers hope to be able to 'turn off' the third copy of the gene and so reverse or eliminate typical features of Down's syndrome, such as problems with cognitive function, memory and speech.

Experiments on mice with Down's syndrome have shown abnormalities in the synapses, or circuits, between nerve cells, leading to the kind of intellectual disability seen in Down's syndrome (and Alzheimer's disease, to which those with Down's syndrome are more prone than the rest of the population).

It may be, for example, that one gene may play a role in intellectual disability by preventing brain chemicals moving into the forebrain. In the future, this gene could be the target for very specific drugs to 'downregulate' or cancel out the action of the extra gene. The theory is that a drug to boost the activity of brain cells could have a marked effect on restoring memory and boosting learning in those with Down's syndrome, though the theory has yet to translate into effective treatments.

5

Diagnosis – antenatal tests

As is well known, Down's syndrome can be diagnosed during pregnancy. A positive result presents a pregnant woman with one of the most difficult situations she can face. Invasive and worrying tests carried out well into pregnancy are still the standard offerings of the medical profession, which has been criticised for allowing technical advances to outstrip the moral issues they raise. So, should you have the tests? Will testing lead to more and more invasive testing? Are you putting your pregnancy at risk? When the tests have been done, what if you emerge as having a very good chance of, or with a definitive diagnosis that you are, carrying a baby with Down's syndrome?

Even if reliable diagnostic testing were available early on in pregnancy, it would solve little or nothing for most mothers as it would still offer no cure for Down's syndrome. Instead, many mothers feel that the tests only leave them with the sole responsibility for the pregnancy and without any real idea of who will help them with that responsibility after the birth.

In the UK, a moral furore was raised by the decision that all pregnant women be offered screening for Down's syndrome. This has been interpreted as eugenics by some. Certainly, the decision doesn't raise any new moral dilemmas – the tests are simply available to more people.

While much research is afoot to pick up markers for Down's syndrome earlier in pregnancy – via blood tests or new scanning techniques – testing for Down's syndrome at any stage of pregnancy remains a moral dilemma. In effect, diagnostic testing for Down's syndrome offers two choices: to continue with the pregnancy with what has been termed the 'dubious gift of knowledge' (Jane Wheatley, writing in *The Times*) or to terminate the pregnancy.

Antenatal testing is just a social euphemism for termination. It is in effect asking you to make a social decision at a highly personal time of your life. People with Down's syndrome are viewed as a burden on society and the most likely outcome of testing has to be termination of the pregnancy in order to lighten that burden.

35

Otherwise, what is the point of testing? Why not test for genes for a propensity to child sex offences, or even alcoholism, both of which do far more damage than harmless children with Down's syndrome. Testing amounts to eugenics because mothers cannot be offered any cure for Down's syndrome – only a decision whether to continue the pregnancy or not.
Tiffany, mother of Jacquie

There are times when I find the burden of care intolerable and feel my own life has gone down the drain. There is never enough funding and support. Forget enough time to yourself. But Jack didn't ask to be born and he is so sweet – looking back, I don't know if I could have had a termination, even if I had known the baby had Down's syndrome, which I didn't.
Ruth, mother of Jack

Having a termination because my baby had Down's syndrome was very hard indeed, but I still think it would have been even harder to bring such a child up. The event marked me profoundly and left me with a grief that I think will be lifelong, but I don't think I could have coped without going to pieces emotionally and spiritually – without my life being ruined, as well as my partner's life and the lives of my two other children, a boy and a girl. Nature ends many pregnancies where there is a genetic mishap, like Down's syndrome. I feel I was a victim of genetic roulette.
Claire

Some women find the idea of testing reassuring as it enables them to know as much as possible about their baby before the birth. Others choose to have no tests, deciding that they will accept their baby, no matter what.

Still others have every test going as a matter of course. Sometimes, perhaps, they do so without having thought through the implications – namely, that one test can lead to another, and then another, and then maybe to a difficult decision at the end of it all as to whether to terminate the pregnancy or not. A major criticism of antenatal testing is the lack of (time-consuming and costly) counselling about its implications and any results.

So, should you have tests?

Four out of five pregnant women opt for screening tests and 95 per cent of those with positive results for abnormalities choose to accept a termination of their pregnancy.

First and foremost, however, you are entitled to refuse tests, including scans, though some women feel obliged to once their doctor has suggested it.

Antenatal testing can be stressful – especially as many women feel more sensitive than usual during pregnancy. You may not want the anxiety that tests can involve – the actual procedure, waiting for the results and receiving the news. On the other hand, many women feel that they would rather know what's what with their baby as far as possible, so that they can prepare themselves for its arrival.

One common myth is that testing invariably leads to termination – some women just want to know. If you do decide on a termination, however, the matter is further complicated by the fact that the test results currently are available so late on in pregnancy that a termination effectively means going through labour. Even if there was an earlier test, it still might not make things much easier. While earlier detection and termination might be less traumatic physically for a mother, who will have had less time to bond with the baby, the distress of it and grief for a lost pregnancy can be just as keenly felt. This grief can be unexpected, especially for women who have no doubt about termination. A common reaction after the event is, 'But no one warned me I'd feel like this.'

There are ongoing emotional effects of testing, mainly in terms of delaying certain emotional and psychological connection with your unborn baby. For example, you may be reluctant to talk about the baby to others or even to think much about it. Some research suggests that women unconsciously do not tune into their baby's movements until after they obtain their test results. It's also natural to feel anxiety, distress, guilt, sadness or depression. On the other hand, some women feel even more anxious and distressed if they don't have the tests and may face an anxious pregnancy until delivery.

In the end, only you can know which option will suit you best. Here are some factors to bear in mind. Testing might be for you if:

- you or your partner need peace of mind and to be assured that your pregnancy and baby are normal

- you want to know if your baby has a problem so as to inform yourself about his or her condition as fully as possible
- you feel you just couldn't cope with a child who is different or who has a problem and would definitely terminate your pregnancy if this were the case.

Testing might not be for you if:

- you could not terminate a pregnancy and are prepared to accept your baby as he or she is
- you couldn't cope with the anxiety and stress of the testing procedure
- you don't feel that it's worth risking miscarriage just to know.

Making an informed decision

If you're not sure, but, for various reasons, feel that there is a good chance of your having a Down's syndrome baby, the following points might help.

- Inform yourself as fully as possible about Down's syndrome so that you're not under false impressions about what the condition does and doesn't involve. Remember that people with Down's syndrome can have fulfilling, quality lives.
- Take time alone to think it through. Decisions do not have to be made in a hurry.
- Discuss it with your partner and any trusted friends.

Genetic counselling

If you have a family history of genetic or congenital conditions, you can ask your GP to refer you for genetic counselling, preferably before you become pregnant. There you will be able to discuss the likelihood of your baby being affected with the same condition and how best to cope. If you are already pregnant, you should still ask to see a doctor, midwife or counsellor with specialist knowledge who can help you think about which tests are best for you.

Antenatal tests

There are two types of antenatal test that can be offered during pregnancy – screening tests and diagnostic tests.

- *Screening tests* estimate the chances of the baby having Down's syndrome. They will only tell you if this is likely or unlikely, not whether you are having a baby with Down's syndrome or not. It is important to realize that screening tests are far from infallible. Most of the mothers deemed to be likely to have a baby with Down's syndrome in fact go on to have babies with no genetic abnormalities.
- *Diagnostic tests* tell whether or not the baby actually has Down's syndrome. It's important to realize that diagnostic tests carry risks (outlined for the different procedures described below). Chief of these is miscarriage. The general figure quoted is that 1 per cent of cases result in miscarriage after amniotic tests. To put it another way, invasive testing causes around 300 miscarriages a year, mostly of healthy babies, according to Professor Kypros Nicolaides at the Harris Bright Research Centre, King's College, London, who adds that statistics show that, for every baby with a disability detected by invasive tests, four healthy babies were lost to miscarriage. (It is also worth remembering that many babies with Down's syndrome miscarry anyway, though it may be easier to accept a miscarriage than a termination.) As well as the possibility of outright loss of the baby, there is also the risk of permanent damage to the unborn baby. Although invasive procedures are carried out while viewing the baby via a scan, there is always the possibility of the needle entering the baby at some vulnerable point. Some people feel that this point is not highlighted enough by doctors, though doctors usually say that the risk of this is slight.

Screening tests

Blood tests

Over the last 20 years, screening tests for chromosomal disorders have become more efficient, though there is still a long way to go. At the moment, the most commonly used form of screening test is one or more blood tests, or maternal serum screening – usually the triple test.

Blood tests – performed at 16–18 weeks of pregnancy – measure levels of certain pregnancy hormones. These are then analysed together with your age to assess your chances of having a child with Down's syndrome.

In the triple test, the mother's blood is checked for three substances – alpha-fetoprotein (AFP), unconjugated oestriol (uE3) and human chorionic gonadotropin (hCG). It is not known why, but, in Down's syndrome, levels of alpha-fetoprotein are more likely to be low than with babies who are developing normally. However, if your test does show low alpha-fetoprotein levels, this doesn't definitively mean that your baby has Down's, only that there is an increased likelihood of it. The level of oestriol is also likely to be lower in a Down's syndrome pregnancy. Levels of human chorionic gonadotropin hormone, on the other hand, are greater in Down's syndrome pregnancies.

The chances of your baby having Down's syndrome are calculated by considering your age and medical history, together with the results of the blood tests. It is also important to be sure of the pregnancy dates (that is, your baby's gestational age) and the dating scan you have can help to establish this.

Results are expressed in differing ways, but often are described as 'screen positive' or 'screen negative'.

- *Screen positive* means your baby has a chance of having Down's syndrome that is more than 1 in 250, though, in fact, the majority of babies who test positive are perfectly healthy. If your blood test is positive, your doctor or midwife will discuss with you whether or not you would like to have further invasive tests.
- *Screen negative* means that your baby has a less than 1 in 250 chance, though you cannot be completely sure that your baby doesn't have Down's from this result alone.

How accurate is the test? It is hard to speak of accuracy in relation to a test that only measures the possibility and isn't diagnostic. Indeed, some doctors feel that the whole procedure is a complete waste of time (see The quadruple test, below). While statistics vary from country to country, around 45 in 1000 pregnancies are shown to have low alpha-fetoprotein levels, but only 1 or 2 of these will be babies born with Down's syndrome or other serious genetic conditions. Statistically speaking, the results of your blood test are far more likely to be negative than positive. A false positive result could worry you needlessly about having a baby with a potentially serious health problem and, indeed, this is the main complaint about this test.

If the result is positive, you may be offered *amniocentesis*. This is where amniotic fluid is drawn from the uterus through a needle around week 16. Another option is *chorionic villius sampling* (CVS), where a sample of the developing placenta is removed around week 11.

The quadruple test

Many doctors believe that a four-stage, or quadruple, test is more effective at detecting Down's syndrome than the triple or double test.

The test looks for levels of four markers for Down's syndrome in the mother's blood. As well as looking for low levels of alpha-fetoprotein and unconjugated oestriol and high levels of human chorionic gonadotropin, this test also measures inhibin – high levels of which also indicate a greater chance of Down's syndrome.

In a study of around 46,000 pregnant mothers, researchers from St Bartholomews Hospital in London and The London School of Medicine and Dentistry found that some women are offered the quadruple test, but that many women miss out, despite it costing little more to do than the double test.

The quadruple test is used across the world, but is not the standard test offered in the UK. In the above study, the quadruple test detected 81 per cent of the pregnancies. The detection rate using maternal age alone, using a cut-off age of 35, was 51 per cent.

Research from the Princess Anne Hospital in Southampton suggests that blood testing is no more effective than scans and that the triple test is unnecessary. Dr David Howe, a consultant in foetal/maternal health, found that the normal mid-pregnancy ultrasound scan can, in many cases, pick out the developing differences between babies with Down's syndrome and others. Also, the research found that the mathematical equations used to calculate the chances and consider a mother's age did not take into account that more women are having babies later in life than previously, so leading to false results.

More effective blood tests in the future

New technology may offer a non-invasive alternative to amniocentesis in a few years time. A method of identifying foetal DNA and other genetic material in the mother's blood has been developed by Dr Dennis Lo and Dr James Wainscoat at the University of Oxford. It is hoped that the blood tests, once available, will provide reliable information as to a number of inherited disorders, including Down's syndrome, replacing amniocentesis and CVS.

Research into more accurate blood tests continues. Researchers at Birmingham Heartlands Hospital have developed a DNA test that cuts the normal diagnosis time from about 15 days to just 1. The test copies tiny amounts of DNA called polymerase chain reaction (PCA), then 'magnifies' them so that any genetic markers associated with Down's syndrome can be recognized.

Tested on 2083 pregnancies, its accuracy rate was almost 100 per cent. However, in this test there were problems separating foetal cells from the mother's blood.

In another study of 4412 women, scientists from the Foundation for Blood Research in Scarborough, Maine, found that blood tests carried out in the first trimester (first three months) of pregnancy picked up more than 60 per cent of 48 babies with Down's syndrome, which were confirmed by amniocentesis or CVS tests. The scientists measured abnormal levels of two proteins – pregnancy-associated protein A and either human chorionic gonadotropin (hCG) or a part of the hormone called hCG-free beta subunit.

Scans

Using ultrasound scans, researchers have looked to several possible signs of Down's syndrome in the unborn baby, including abnormalities of the heart, bowel and kidneys, to provide the keys to diagnosis. However, many of these remain controversial – they are not definitive and can also be found in typical unborn babies.

More definite are scans that look at two specific areas of the baby's body have proved helpful. The *nuchal scan* looks at the back of the neck, while the newer *nasal scan* examines a bone in the baby's nose (this is explained below). They were both pioneered by Professor Kypros Nicolaides at the Harris Bright Research Centre, King's College, London. He believes that widespread use of these methods could drastically cut down on invasive diagnostic testing, such as amniocentesis. For example, if doctors spent an extra few seconds checking for the nasal bone during routine scans, Professor Nicolaides estimates that this would reduce the number of invasive tests from 30,000 to 10,000. Some doctors in the UK and USA are using nuchal and nasal scans in combination with other tests.

Nuchal scan

The *nuchal translucency ultrasound test* is a sophisticated scanning technique that measures the skin at the back of the unborn baby's neck, looking for fluid. A normal nuchal translucency thickness ranges from 1 to 2 millimetres and varies with the age of the unborn baby. Abnormal swelling may be a sign of Down's syndrome.

Professor Nicolaides was inspired to develop this method by Dr John Langdon Haydon Down's original description of the syndrome in 1866, when he observed that the skin of affected people seemed too big for their bodies.

Performed at around 11 weeks of pregnancy, this is a screening test that, like other screening tests, assesses the likelihood of your baby having Down's syndrome. It is also a possible marker for other problems and genetic syndromes, as heart defects and lymphatic development also cause abnormal swelling in the necks of unborn babies. What happens is that the back of your baby's neck is screened closely and the layer of fluid between the two folds of skin (the nuchal folds) is measured. A thicker layer of fluid than normal means that there is a chance that your baby has Down's syndrome.

Like other scans, it is quite painless, though you can feel somewhat uncomfortable as you need a full bladder in order to push the womb up out of your pelvis, so that the baby can be seen clearly.

Depending on the outcome, your baby will be assessed as having a greater or lesser chance of having Down's, though most babies deemed to have a greater chance of it are in fact later found not to have Down's. The test is more reliable in the hands of an experienced operator. Your chances are assessed in combination with other risk factors, including your age and results of blood tests. Depending on the outcome, you can choose to go on to have other diagnostic tests, such as chorionic villus sampling or amniocentesis (see below).

Nasal scan

This new scanning technique is another non-invasive method that could give a more accurate idea as to whether or not a baby is affected by Down's syndrome. It has been shown to have a 93 per cent detection rate. It involves the simple procedure of checking for a bone in the baby's nose.

Down noted that affected babies had small noses with a flat bridge. Professor Nicolaides found that the majority of them – 73 per cent – are actually lacking a bone, as opposed to typical babies, where the figure is just 0.5–1 per cent. If the nose bone is present, then the chances of having a baby with Down's syndrome are automatically reduced to one-third of the results of other tests, according to Professor Nicolaides.

Nicolaides' research looked at 701 pregnant women considered to be likely to have babies with Down's syndrome due to their age and nuchal scan results. The women had a scan between 11 and 14 weeks to examine the babies' profiles and it was found that the nasal bone was underdeveloped in 61.8 per cent of the babies with Down's syndrome, but in only 1.2 per cent of babies who were developing normally. No other available tests approach the ability of the nasal scan to detect Down's syndrome, Nicolaides believes. This is because, in a scan, the bone shows up clearly as white, whereas its absence shows as blackness – in other words, it is pretty clear whether or not the bone is present. The combination of nasal bone screening with other tests for Down's syndrome may identify the disorder in more than 98 per cent of babies, according to Professor Nicolaides.

Diagnostic tests

Amniocentesis

This involves a fine needle being passed into the womb, using an ultrasound scan to guide it, and taking a sample of the amniotic fluid around the baby. It's done under local anaesthetic. This fluid, which contains fetal cells that can be examined for chromosome tests, is then analysed and certain biochemical, chromosomal or neural tube defects can be identified. Results may take two to four weeks to come. Down's syndrome can be diagnosed at about 15–16 weeks by amniocentesis. There is a risk of about 1 in 100–200 of a spontaneous miscarriage occurring after the test.

Amniocentesis is usually carried out between weeks 14 and 18 of pregnancy; some doctors may do them as early as week 13. Side-effects the mother might experience include cramping, bleeding, infection and leaking of amniotic fluid afterwards. There is a slight increase in the risk of miscarriage if you have the test – the normal rate of miscarriage at this time of pregnancy is 2 to 3 per cent and amniocentesis increases that risk by an additional 0.5 to 1 per cent. However, many fetuses with Down's syndrome miscarry spontaneously around this point in the pregnancy or afterwards.

Chorionic villus sampling (CVS)

CVS can be performed at 10–12 weeks – earlier than amniocentesis. Results are available within two weeks.

Instead of amniotic fluid being taken, a small amount of tissue from the chorionic villi (tiny, finger-like fronds on the placenta) is removed (also called the chorionic layer). These cells contain genetic material that is identical to that found in the baby and this can be analysed to reveal the chromosomal make-up (and sex) of your baby. The cells can be collected in the same way as for amniocentesis, also with the guidance of ultrasound, but another method is to insert a catheter into the uterus through the vagina or abdominal wall. The method used depends on the position of the placenta or your doctor's personal preference.

Side-effects experienced by the mother are the same as for amniocentesis (see above). The risk of miscarriage after CVS is slightly higher than for amniocentesis, increasing the normal risk of miscarriage to 3 to 5 per cent. Studies have shown that the more experienced the doctor performing the CVS, the lower the rate of miscarriage. Early on in the use of CVS, a number of babies were identified with missing or shortened fingers or toes. However, that has been connected to the use of CVS before the week 10 of pregnancy.

Fetoscopy

Largely superseded by scans, fetoscopy is now rarely performed.

The mother and baby are both sedated and an endoscope is fed through the abdominal wall into the uterus. A needle is then inserted through the endoscope tube. This method allows samples of the baby's blood, liver or skin to be taken.

The advantages of fetoscopy are that the unborn baby can be seen and its tissue and blood sampled. Also, treatment, such as blood transfusion, may be given.

If your baby does have Down's syndrome

Do not rush into any decision – take a few days to think things over and discuss them with your partner. No matter what advice you receive – from doctors, family, friends – any decisions you make about your pregnancy do not have to be made on the spot. It can be very helpful to allow space for thoughts to emerge that are by no means obvious while you are experiencing the first shock of receiving the news. You may also find it helpful to see if you can receive counselling – preferably counselling that gives you access to as wide a range of information as possible and the chance to make an informed decision based on facts about Down's syndrome today. It can also be very beneficial to meet a family with a child who has Down's syndrome, either via your medical carers or a support group, such as the Down's Syndrome Association in the UK.

It is worth repeating that you should give yourself time to come to terms with your feelings. It is not an easy experience to deal with and your emotions are likely to be on a roller coaster, especially as pregnancy hormones can play havoc with your moods at the best of times. This is probably not what you hoped for from your pregnancy and, with the best will in the world, takes a great deal of adjusting to. Chapter 1 of this book looked at how some new mothers reacted to the news that their baby had Down's syndrome. While they found this out after delivery, their emotions, connected with shock and grieving, are likely to be similar to yours – disbelief, anger and the question 'Why me?' Do try to find someone strong, warm and trustworthy with whom to share the negative emotions that may be tearing you apart.

6

Health issues

Many children with Down's syndrome are fit and healthy, needing the same kind of general medical care as any other child, with your family doctor providing routine healthcare and immunizations. However, some health conditions requiring more care are more common in children with Down's syndrome than other children. The most serious of these, which nearly half of them have, is congenital heart defects. These may require heart surgery and ongoing care. Children with Down's syndrome also have a greater tendency to succumb to infections than other children, particularly chest and sinus infections. Babies may also have problems regulating their temperature and can have very dry skin. Chapter 9 looks at what you can do to boost your child's immune system and general health.

This chapter outlines health problems that tend to be more common in children with Down's syndrome. Set out all together like this, it's a pretty daunting list. As one mother put it, 'You could never imagine there was so much going on in one little body', but your child is highly unlikely to have them all and may even not have any. While certain health conditions are more common in children with Down's syndrome, these problems are far from inevitable and are almost always treatable, allowing the vast majority of those with Down's syndrome to enjoy good health. Thanks to modern medicine, most children with Down's syndrome can lead healthy lives.

I feel very strongly that parents should trust their intuition and insist on a proper diagnosis if they feel that something is wrong. I spent three and a half years being sent round the houses with Luke before he was eventually diagnosed with reflux [gastro-oesophageal reflux disease, the symptoms of which include vomiting and reluctance to feed, is caused by a weak valve or sphincter at the top of the stomach so that feeds come back up into the oesophagus, causing acid and pain, instead of being digested; see p. 53 for more. It was just a tiny gurgling sound in his tummy that alerted me from when he was only a few weeks old, but no one would listen to me when I described the

symptoms. Unfortunately, although the reflux has now been treated after major surgery, Luke has learned to associate feeding with pain and has been left with a massive eating disorder that I feel we may be tackling for several years to come.
Jo, mother of Luke, 6

Getting medical help

Unfortunately it is beyond the scope of this book to look at medical problems in great detail. These can be idiosyncratic in children with Down's syndrome, who may sometimes have multiple conditions to contend with. The Useful addresses section at the back of the book contains contact details for further information on many conditions.

Meanwhile, do mention any concerns you may have to your doctor – don't put them down to just being part of Down's syndrome and don't allow medical professionals to do so either. It's also worth pointing out that children with Down's syndrome are just as likely as any other child to develop a health problem that has absolutely nothing to do with the syndrome at all.

In a survey of 1500 people by the Down's Syndrome Association (DSA) in the UK, it was found that 72 per cent were satisfied with the quality of healthcare provision they received, while 28 per cent reported a high level of dissatisfaction. It appears that, while attitudes have improved, levels of medical support for those with learning disabilities may vary.

The DSA, together with the Down's Syndrome Medical Interest Group (DSMIG), has produced healthcare guidelines to assist families and health professionals in setting up screening programmes so that health problems can be picked up early on and treated before they become more serious. The DSA is also working hard to improve the situation in other ways, such as training health professionals, maintaining a website specifically for health professionals on learning disability and campaigning for changes.

Getting the best from your medical carers

Finding out as much as possible about your child's condition is vital for many parents who seek to come to terms with the reality of caring for their child.

Don't hesitate to ask doctors and other medical professionals for explanations of words or procedures that are new to you. It need only take a minute or so for them to explain and they should be happy to do so. For regular appointments, it can help to write down a list of concerns or questions that you want to ask, prioritizing them in order of importance. File the answers away, together with any written reports on your child from doctors, therapists and others.

Heart defects

Some families find that the issue of Down's syndrome pales into insignificance beside the life and overall health of their child as they face the impact of a dual diagnosis, such as Down's syndrome and a heart defect.

Up to 45 per cent of children with Down's syndrome have congenital heart defects. The most common defects are *atrioventricular septal defect*, *persistent ductus arteriosus* and *tetralogy of Fallot*.

- *Atrioventricular septal defect* occurs when tissue fails to come together in the heart while the baby is forming in the womb, resulting in a hole or holes in the top chambers of the heart as well as valve abnormalities. This is the most common heart defect in children with Down's syndrome, occuring in nearly 60 per cent of those born with heart troubles.
- *Persistent ductus arteriosus* is when a channel between the pulmonary artery and the aorta fails to close in the baby's first day of life, resulting in an increased flow of blood into the lungs.
- *Tetralogy of Fallot* is a complicated group of congenital heart defects, including a ventricular septal defect, which allows blood to pass from the right ventricle to the left ventricle without going through the lungs, a stenosis (narrowing) at or just beneath the

pulmonary valve, so partially blocking the flow of blood from the right ventricle to the lungs, as well as an aorta in an abnormal position. All this means that blood flow into the lungs is obstructed, which results in cyanosis (bluish discoloration of the skin due to poor blood oxygenation) that may be noticeable when the baby is crying, feeding or at other times.

In the first few months, signs of heart defects may include rapid breathing and failure to grow and gain weight. The situation is complicated, however, by the fact that children may show these signs without having heart trouble and some children may have heart problems yet have no obvious symptoms. Because of this, it is usually recommended that an echocardiogram be performed on all newborns with Down's syndrome. Early screening is all the more vital anyway as some heart defects need to be treated by the time the child is six months old. (If your child is older and has never had an echocardiogram, ask your doctor about having one.)

Learning of a heart condition can be another serious blow to parents who are already coming to terms with the news of Down's syndrome. If surgery is recommended, there may be a very painful period of suspense during which some parents feel that they hardly dare bond with their baby. When surgery is not possible, the suspense is more painful and likely to be prolonged. It may help to talk to someone in the same position. The Down's Heart Group in the UK offers support and information to families who have a member with Down's syndrome and congenital heart defects (see the Useful addresses section at the back of the book for contact details).

Most heart defects in children with Down's syndrome can be surgically corrected and improvements in surgery have made a great difference to the life expectancy and quality of life for people with Down's syndrome.

Leukaemia and cancer

Children with Down's syndrome have a greater risk of developing a type of leukaemia called *acute myeloid leukaemia*, which affects roughly 1 in 50–100 children with Down's syndrome, especially in the first three years of life. The good news is that children with Down's syndrome respond well to treatment and have a high cure rate.

Other types of leukaemia, including *chronic myeloid leukaemia* and *chronic lymphatic leukaemia* seem to be less common in children with Down's syndrome than other children.

A form of leukaemia called *transient myeloproliferative syndrome* or *transient abnormal myelopoiesis* (TAM) is also seen in newborns. It's hardly ever seen in children unless they have Down's syndrome and, as the name suggests, this curious kind of leukaemia often disappears without treatment. However, for unknown reasons (possibly genetic), in about 20 to 30 per cent of cases, full-blown leukaemia will develop – usually acute myeloid leukaemia. The treatment for children with Down's syndrome who have leukaemia is largely the same as for other children, though an extra-careful watch will be kept for infection and heart problems.

Overall, though, people with Down's syndrome have a much lower risk of developing cancer than the rest of the population. The reason for this is not really known, though there are differing theories. One is that the extra chromosome 21 may contain genes that suppress the development of tumours or slow the replication (reproduction or duplication) of cancer cells as this chromosome is known to play an important part in the immune system. Another theory is that people with Down's syndrome are less often exposed to environmental factors that could cause cancer, such as smoking.

Down's – the key to lung cancer protection?

Scientists have speculated that people with Down's syndrome could show the way forward in terms of lung cancer protection.

Research at the School of Pharmacy, London University, suggests that a gene called USP25 may be part of a protective mechanism the body has that stops us from developing lung cancer. While those with Down's syndrome have three copies of this gene and have a low propensity to develop lung cancer, it is often missing from the cancer cells of people who have lung cancer. The gene is similar to others that are known to have protective effects in relation to cancer. Although research is in its early stages, it is thought that understanding more about this gene could show the way forward in terms of more general cancer protection.

Digestive problems

These also tend to be more common in children with Down's syndrome than other children and may show up dramatically after birth or develop slowly. If your baby is having persistent trouble, ask for a thorough medical check.

Symptoms of gastrointestinal trouble include:

- failure to feed
- vomiting
- diarrhoea
- constipation
- poor weight gain (though this last is a feature of Down's syndrome anyway).

Constipation is common in children with Down's syndrome, believed to be because of low muscle tone, poor mobility, diet and inadequate fluid intake. More exercise, extra fluid, fruit and cereals may solve the problem, but, if not, your doctor can prescribe a laxative. If, however, the constipation persists, other causes should be considered, including an underactive thyroid (hypothyroidism) and Hirschsprung's disease. Both of these conditions can cause constipation and are more common in those with Down's syndrome than in the general population.

Hirschsprung's disease is an abnormality of the large bowel, whereby part of the bowel wall has nerve cells missing so that it is less effective at moving stools along to the anus. Symptoms are:

- failure to pass stools
- chronic constipation
- poor weight gain
- vomiting
- a swollen tummy.

Treatment usually involves surgery to remove the abnormal part of the bowel.

Structural problems affect some 10 per cent of children with Down's syndrome and are often picked up at birth. These include small bowel obstruction, when food cannot pass from the stomach to the large bowel, a similar problem with the pancreas and narrowing or blockage of the anus. Treatment is usually in the form of surgery.

Gastro-oesophageal reflux is when food comes back from the stomach up into the oesophagus, often because the muscle at the top of the stomach is immature and the stomach muscles are less effective than they should be. Symptoms are discomfort, especially after feeding, and projectile vomiting. Medication can often sort this one out, while feeding the baby upright and allowing plenty of time to bring up wind can also help. Occasionally surgery is used to tighten the join between the oesophagus and the stomach.

Some children suffer from malabsorption, which is when their bodies are unable to absorb the nutrients from food. The main type of malabsorption affecting children with Down's syndrome is coeliac disease, which is an allergy to gluten, found in wheat and other cereal grains. Symptoms include:

- poor growth
- abnormal stools (bulky or frothy)
- diarrhoea
- swollen tummy
- tiredness and irritability.

Treatment is a gluten-free diet, followed under medical supervision.

Thyroid problems

Part of the classic image of people with Down's syndrome is a tendency to be sluggish. It is now appreciated that this can be contributed to by poor functioning of the thyroid, which may affect some 10 per cent of children, but 30–50 per cent of adults. Screening for thyroid dysfunction is especially important for children under three, as correct thyroid function is vital to brain development.

Hypothyroidism results from a malfunctioning thyroid gland, which produces too little of the hormone thyroxin, which helps brain growth and other body tissue. It is the most common endocrinological problem in children with Down's syndrome. Signs of hypothyroidism include an enlarged tongue, constipation and poor circulation, but these are also found in children who don't have thyroid problems, so testing is very important.

Hyperthyroidism is when the thyroid gland is overactive, causing swelling in the neck, abnormal sweating and a rapid pulse rate.

Thyroid problems are easily treated with medication.

Diabetes

Like thyroid problems, diabetes is an endocrinological disorder. Both are auto-immune diseases, which is when the body produces antibodies that destroy or overstimulate vital tissues. In some cases, the two conditions coexist in children with Down's syndrome.

Diabetes, usually of Type 1, or insulin-dependent, form is more common in children with Down's syndrome than other children. Estimates vary, but, in some areas, it may exist in as many as 15 per cent of children with Down's syndrome. Whether or not obesity in later life is linked with Type 2 diabetes has not been conclusively proved, but is worth keeping in mind.

Diabetes can, in some cases, be controlled by diet alone – lowering intakes of sugar, fat and starch (especially important for children with Down's syndrome, who have a tendency to be overweight). Alternatively, insulin may be given.

Symptoms of diabetes include:

- excessive thirst
- frequent and/or increased urination
- an odd, sweetish or fruity smell to your child's breath
- weight loss
- listlessness.

Do consult your doctor if you fear the presence of diabetes. Early diagnosis is vital in order to prevent its well-known complications, which include stroke, heart attack, as well as problems with the eyes, kidneys and feet.

Hearing loss

Some 60–80 per cent of children with Down's syndrome have hearing problems. They may have been born with them or acquired them due to ear infections and a resulting build-up of fluid in the ear (otitis media). Smaller than normal ear canals may play a part in a child's hearing difficulties. Sinusitis and increased levels of ear wax may also cause problems.

Hearing loss may cause some behavioural problems in your child as a result of becoming frustrated because he or she cannot hear. Some children switch off and don't bother to try and listen, so, unless the hearing problem is picked up, it is easy to blame this on the child's personality or on Down's syndrome itself. To make matters even more confusing, if your child has glue ear, how much can be heard will vary depending on how much fluid is in the ears at any one time.

A constant mild hearing loss can affect the child's ability to perceive the differences between some consonant sounds such as 'b's and 'p's, plural endings ('s' sounds). So, while he or she may understand short, simple sentences, longer ones may cause confusion.

The impact of all this on the child's language development will be obvious. So, don't simply assume that all language delay relates to Down's syndrome. Regular hearing tests are important.

Immunizations

In the light of the furore over the MMR (measles, mumps, rubella) vaccine and its supposed links with autism, you may well be undecided as to whether or not your child should be vaccinated.

Current recommendations by the Down Syndrome Medical Interest Group (DSMIG) are that children with Down's syndrome can be offered all routine immunizations and, due to their greater propensity towards infection, maybe extra ones, too, such as flu jabs. There is currently no evidence that vaccines, including MMR, are likely to cause an adverse reaction in children with Down's syndrome. The diseases that MMR protects against would be likely to be serious for a child with the syndrome, say the DSMIG.

Eye problems

Your child's ability to see is not affected by the characteristic slanting eye shape or epicanthic folds associated with Down's syndrome. However, some children with Down's syndrome do have more eye problems than other children. For example, up to 3 per cent of babies with Down's syndrome have cataracts, which is when opacity or cloudiness of the lens in the eye restricts the passage of light into the eyeball. This can easily be corrected surgically. Glasses or contact lenses may also be used later in life.

Other possible eye problems include myopia, short-sightedness.

This is found in around 14 per cent of preschool children with Down's syndrome. Hypermytropia – long-sightedness – affects some 40 per cent of preschool children with Down's syndrome, who also often have a squint. Astigmatism, which is a problem with focusing, affects about 30 per cent of children with Down's syndrome.

Nystagmus – involuntary eye movements – are experienced by 10 per cent of children with Down's syndrome.

Strabismus, which is the term for a squint or any misalignment of the eyes, affects 20 per cent of children with Down's syndrome. Such problems can be corrected by glasses or, in more severe cases, surgery.

Eye infections, treatable with antibiotic drops or ointment, also tend to be more commonly experienced by children with Down's syndrome than other children. This is due to the narrow tear ducts, which can become easily blocked. Conjunctivitis is a very common condition, involving inflammation of the conjunctiva – the membrane that lines the eyelid – resulting in redness, irritation and discharge. Your doctor can prescribe drops, cream or ointment.

Blepharitis, which is inflammation of the skin around the eyelashes, often coexists with general dry skin. It may help to wipe the lids with cooled boiled water, adding sodium bicarbonate (a teaspoon per 570 ml/1 pint of water) or very diluted baby shampoo in more severe cases.

Keratoconus does not usually develop before young adulthood. This is characterized by the cornea bulging outwards and becoming cone-shaped. Contact lenses can help to prevent this process continuing.

Your child may benefit from specialized care. If this is the case, your doctor can refer him or her to an eye specialist, such as an orthoptist or ophthalmologist.

When should my child have eye tests?

If you notice a squint, ask your family doctor to refer your child for an eye test as soon as possible. For children who don't have any obvious eye problems, screening by an orthoptist is recommended between 1 year and 18 months and again at the age of 4 years, prior to starting school, in addition to routine developmental checks.

Glasses

If your child has to wear glasses, try to associate them with fun activities, such as looking at books or playing activity games, suggests Barbara Crofts, associate specialist in ophthalmology at the Oxford Eye Hospital. If you yourself wear glasses, try to wear them more of the time. Enlisting the support of nursery school teachers and playgroup leaders in this can also be helpful.

Ensure that the glasses fit comfortably and don't dig into your child's head. Your child's small nose makes glasses more liable to slide down than usual, so do return to the optician for refitting and adjusting if necessary. Once your child realizes that the glasses help him or her see better, he or she is likely to want to wear them.

Skeletal problems

Approximately 15 per cent of people with Down's syndrome have *atlantoaxial instability*, which is when the first two neck bones are not well aligned because of the presence of loose ligaments. As in most cases there are no symptoms, X-rays are needed to reveal whether or not your child has this. It is important that this is diagnosed because of the risk of injury to the neck and spine if the child later engages in sport. A child who does have this may need to choose physical activities carefully, avoiding certain more vigorous sports, such as football, gymnastics and diving. However, it is unnecessary to eliminate all exercise In some cases, surgery may help.

Other conditions can include looseness or dislocations in the hip and knee. These problems are usually treated surgically.

Flat feet are also common, which can lead to bunions, callouses and sprains. Your child may need orthopedic supports in comfortable shoes.

Epilepsy

Around 5 to 10 per cent of those with Down's syndrome also have epilepsy, due to different types of chromosomal abnormality. Brainwave abnormalities have also been picked up by electro-encephalogram (EEG) in around 25 per cent of those with Down's syndrome.

Types of epilepsy that seem to be more common in those with Down's syndrome than is generally the case include *infantile spasms* in the first year of life and, more often, *tonic-clonic* or *myoclonic* (generalized seizures that involve the whole brain). Tonic-clonic seizures involve loss of consciousness, while myoclonic ones may consist of brief muscle contractions or jerking. Another type is *febrile seizures*, which occur due to a high temperature in a young child.

However, epilepsy is rarer in those with Down's syndrome than it is in those with other developmental conditions. One study found that the rate of epilepsy was 6 per cent in a group of people with Down's syndrome, but 18 per cent in another group of mentally retarded people without Down's syndrome.

It should be noted that some conditions can mimic epileptic seizures in those with Down's syndrome. For example, fainting due to heart trouble or the sudden jerky, movements and noises made during sleep apnoea. Sleep deprivation can also worsen existing seizures. For a proper diagnosis, you need to see a neurologist specializing in epilepsy.

Autism and Down's syndrome

An estimated 10 per cent of people with Down's syndrome may also have some form of autistic spectrum disorder, though exact figures are hard to obtain – especially as many cases probably go undiagnosed.

Unlike Down's syndrome, there is no uniform set of clinical features or tests for autism. Telltale signs, however, may include:

- autistic aloneness – preferring to be left alone and not wanting to be held or cuddled
- obsessive desire for sameness – being very upset by changes in daily routines
- lack of eye contact
- odd, repetitive, stereotypical behaviour, such as tapping, spinning, rocking or repetitive play.

Alzheimer's disease

While Alzheimer's disease will hardly be a problem for a newborn baby or young child, there has been a lot of publicity about its links with Down's syndrome and so it is a subject that can worry parents.

Alzheimer's – a degenerative neurological disorder characterized by progressive memory loss, personality deterioration and loss of motor abilities – is around three to five times more common in people with Down's syndrome than in the general population.

The brains of people with Down's syndrome may start showing clinical signs of Alzheimer's when they are in their thirties or sometimes earlier. Usually, Alzheimer's disease doesn't develop before the age of 50.

Exactly why this is the case isn't known. Current research is investigating how certain genes on chromosome 21 may predispose individuals with Down's syndrome to Alzheimer's disease. Meanwhile, some feel that any brain degeneration in those threatened with Alzheimer's may be slowed, or even prevented, by a super-healthy diet supplemented with vitamins and minerals, given from earliest childhood. (See Chapter 9 for more on diet.)

Sleep apnoea

At least 30 per cent (though figures vary and some estimates are of 50 per cent or more) of children with Down's syndrome suffer from *sleep apnoea* – when breathing ceases for ten seconds or more during sleep – due to smaller airway sizes, enlarged adenoids and tonsils and lack of muscle tone, including that of the throat muscles.

Obstructive sleep apnoea – the most common form – occurs when tissues in the upper throat (or airway) collapse at intervals during sleep, thereby blocking the passage of air. Symptoms include snoring, restless sleep and unusual sleeping positions.

Left untreated, sleep apnoea can cause daytime sleepiness and affect behaviour and concentration, exacerbating any developmental delay. Later in life, health risks are thought to include high blood pressure, heart attack and stroke.

Ask your doctor about treatment, which may include referral to a sleep clinic and/or to an ear, nose and throat or other respiratory specialist. See also Chapter 7 for more on sleep problems.

Down's life expectancy doubles

Modern medical care means that people with Down's syndrome are living much longer now than ever before. Life expectancy is currently put at 55–65, and many people with Down's syndrome live longer than that.

The life expectancy of people with Down's syndrome has doubled since the early 1980s, an American study has found. The Centers for Disease Control and Prevention in Atlanta examined death certificates of around 17,900 people with Down's syndrome who died between 1983 and 1997. It was found that, during this period, the average age at death increased from 25 to 49 years. People from non-white races were more likely to die younger than white people with Down's syndrome. Also, people with Down's syndrome were more likely to die from conditions such as congenital heart defects, dementia and leukaemia than the rest of the population.

Preparing for hospital

If your child does have to go into hospital at any time, he or she – like all children – will benefit from being as prepared as possible.

The hospital may well offer you and your child a tour, but, if not, contact the ward your child will stay in and ask if it is possible to be shown round, meet staff and learn more about the medical procedures involved in your child's treatment.

At the same time, ask whether or not it is possible to stay with your child until he or she goes under the anaesthetic and other such options. Most hospitals these days have sleepover facilities for parents, so these could be checked out, too.

You may also find it helpful to talk to other parents whose children have had surgery at the same hospital – ward staff may be able to put you in touch with someone.

Depending on your child's level of understanding, talk as honestly as possible about why he or she needs to go into hospital, emphasizing that it is so the doctor can make him or her better. It may help to use props, such as toy medical kit, dolls, drawings or books. Explain that you will be there, too. If possible, give your child opportunities to play out or discuss events afterwards.

7

Settling down with your new baby

With Freddie, we decided that we would blaze a trail. We were determined that Down's syndrome would make no difference and that Freddie would have access to the widest possible range of opportunities and experiences. It took us quite some time to realize that, far from blazing a trail, we were actually following quite a well-tracked path and that others had been there before us!
Annabel

I remember the health visitor came to see us on the sixth day. I'd been keeping close to home as I was terrified of Tara getting an infection. I asked the health visitor if I could take the baby out. She looked at her and said, very coolly and sweetly, 'Of course. She will love the fresh air.' I think that was the turning point for me in coming to terms with the baby as she was and realizing that she was a tiny person who would enjoy and benefit from new experiences. I couldn't wait to get going after that.
Moira

As with any new baby, there is a period of adjustment as you get to know your little one and evolve some kind of routine at home. Like Annabel and Moira, sooner or later, many mothers just want to get on with it and are determined to integrate the baby into the family and by no means to restrict the rest of the family's activities just because the baby has Down's syndrome. Some mothers do take longer to adapt than others – one reported that her child was four before she felt truly comfortable and unselfconscious about taking him out.

Meanwhile, you are not merely adapting to Down's syndrome, but also to new parenthood. Whether it's your first or fourth baby, it takes time to adjust to the change in the family made by a new person. Give yourself as much time as you need for this, whether it's days, weeks or months.

There is a perception that many babies with Down's syndrome are very 'good' – placid, sleepy and easy to care for, but most newborns spend the majority of their time sleeping and enjoy feeding! Others may be more 'difficult' in terms of crying and settling.

One particular area of difficulty can be breastfeeding. To put it into perspective, this is something that many new mothers find problematic and surveys show that British breastfeeding rates are among the lowest in Europe. Only 7 out of 10 babies receive any breastmilk and this falls to 55 per cent once the baby is a week old. Perseverance can usually lead to successful breastfeeding and the benefits are definitely worthwhile. If you've tried and really can't manage it, enjoy feeding time with your baby nonetheless and you have nothing to feel guilty about.

In these early weeks, concentrate on your baby and yourself – try not to worry about anything else. With regard to your feelings, do be alert for depression, which may take the form of acute tiredness, weepiness and feeling unable to cope. While you may be going through a massive adaptation as you adjust to parenthood and the reality of your baby with Down's syndrome, there is a line between healthy struggle and grief, and being swamped by your emotions (see Chapter 1 for more on post-natal depression and the Useful addresses section for contact details of an organization that can help).

Adapting to parenthood will be easier if you don't expect too much of yourself. Lack of sleep is a major issue for new parents, so try to get enough rest – sleep when your baby sleeps if at all possible. Be disciplined in this – ignore the housework, leave the answerphone on, even leave a 'Please don't disturb' sign on your front door when you're resting. Alternatively, ask a friend or family member to look after your baby while you rest or sleep. If you can't catnap, practise relaxation techniques, have a warm bath or just curl up with a book or in front of the TV.

If possible, share the night feeds with your partner. If you're breastfeeding, try expressing your breast milk into a bottle or perhaps he could make you a warm drink, change a nappy or at least fetch you the baby.

Do accept all offers of help, whether it's cooking a meal, putting a wash on or popping out for some milk. Limit visitors, if need be, or ask your partner to help space them out – don't feel you have to play host to them.

Eat as well as you can and, if you've no time to cook, stock up on nutritious snacks, such as fruit, dried fruit, nuts, milk and wholemeal bread.

If your baby has to stay in hospital

If your baby is poorly and has to spend some time in hospital at first, he or she may sleep much of the time, so you may feel that there isn't much you can do. However, there are vital ways in which you can contribute.

- Cuddle your baby when you can. Babies who are cuddled skin to skin have been shown to gain weight more quickly than babies who spend most of their time in the special care cot. Your baby thrives on your warmth, the sound of your heartbeat and your scent.
- Keep up your breastmilk by expressing it so that your baby can take it by syringe, tube, cup or bottle. Breastmilk will help your baby to thrive and give protection against infection.
- Talk and sing to your baby quietly. He or she can recognize your voice, and that of your partner, remembering from when in the womb, and enjoys hearing them from birth.

The extra benefits of breastfeeding

Breastfeeding gets any baby off to a good start in life, but has extra special benefits when you have a baby with Down's syndrome as it helps develop his or her potential better than is possible with bottlefeeding. Because breastfeeding helps develop the muscles in your baby's face and jaw, it improves mouth and tongue coordination, so helping lessen any future speech problems. As with all babies, breastfeeding also gives protection against infection – especially important for your baby as babies with Down's syndrome are more prone to this. Breastfed babies are reported to have fewer stomach upsets, respiratory tract infections, ear infections and urinary tract infections. Your milk also helps protect against bowel problems, which are more likely in a baby with Down's syndrome. Breastfed babies are less likely to become obese, suffer from constipation or vomiting or develop allergies or diabetes.

Breastmilk contains substances that help the development of babies' brains, retinas, gut lining and the protective sheath for the central nervous system, boosting their overall growth and development.

As with any baby, breastfeeding is a lovely way to get to know your baby and bond with him or her. Your baby will love being held and cuddled while feeding, skin to skin if possible.

Overcoming difficulties

Because most babies with Down's syndrome have low muscle tone (hypotonia), this can make breastfeeding more difficult than usual – your baby may have difficulties coordinating sucking and swallowing, for example. As the tongue is flat, your baby may also have some difficulty positioning it on the breast, with the result that the milk slides to the sides of the mouth rather than being immediately swallowed. This means that your baby has to work harder and longer for less milk, which may well mean that feeding takes longer than usual. Some babies are born prematurely, which can mean that they have more problems breastfeeding than those born around their due dates.

Many babies with Down's syndrome are placid and sleepy in the early weeks. This may mean that you have to set regular feeding times every two to three hours, rather than let your baby decide when to feed, so that he or she has enough milk. Aim for little and often – the norm anyway with many breastfed babies – and try to feed for ten minutes minimum. Try to ensure, too, that your baby empties one breast before starting on the other as the hindmilk, which comes at the end of a feed, is rich in fat and best for the baby who needs to put on weight. At the next feed, start with the other breast and so on to avoid discomfort and the possibility of mastitis.

Support your baby, using cushions if necessary to position him or her well so you're both comfortable. A nursing pillow can help you prop your baby up (it will also help him or her to see around and explore the surroundings and, later, you can use it to support your baby while he or she is learning to sit or play with toys). Your baby should be fairly upright to get the maximum amount of milk from the breast. This is especially important if he or she has any instability in the neck joints. In this case, giving a little extra support with your hand at his or her jaw and chin will help.

Give your baby plenty of opportunities to bring up wind at points during feeding and afterwards. To do this, sit him or her upright, support the head and wait. If nothing happens, rub or pat the baby's back gently.

As your baby grows, muscle tone improves and so breastfeeding will get easier.

Do get support if you are having problems – initially from hospital staff or health visitors or else self-help organizations such as La Lèche League (see the Useful addresses section at the back of the book for contact details). You could also ask medical professionals about specialist feeding therapists or speech and language therapists who may also be able to help. This is because the muscles used in feeding are the same ones as will be used for speech, so early therapy can be very helpful (for more on this, see Chapter 8).

Weight gain

Some babies with Down's syndrome need careful watching to make sure that they gain enough weight. This is especially true if your baby has heart defects, as he or she may well burn up energy faster than do other babies. According to one study, children with congenital heart defects who received any breastfeeding, even when supplemented with bottled milk, had shorter hospital stays and gained weight more easily than babies who were exclusively bottlefed.

Apart from regular weighings, one day-to-day way to monitor weight gain is to keep track of wet nappies. A healthy baby should get through around five or six (disposable) nappies a day. Frequent bowel movements – two to five a day for the first six weeks – are also good signs that your baby is getting enough milk.

If your baby isn't gaining enough weight, despite frequent feeds, try to ensure that he or she is fully awake while feeding. A sleepy baby may need a little extra prodding to ensure that he or she actively sucks all the milk needed, especially to access the richer hindmilk at the end of a feed. Short, frequent feeds may help, as may tactile stimulation, such as hugs, massage or games such as walking your fingers up your baby's arm.

Some early symptoms of a heart problem, such as inadequate weight gain and lack of energy, can be mistaken by parents and professionals as just being characteristic of Down's syndrome itself. While your baby should have been thoroughly checked for heart disease, don't hesitate to mention any concerns to your doctor.

Supplementing breastfeeding

With the best will in the world, breastfeeding alone may not work for everyone or for ever. If your baby isn't gaining enough weight or if you find the whole process just too draining or too much work, there may come a time when you want to supplement, either by expressing your own milk into bottles or giving bottled milk. Don't feel guilty about this, especially if you decide to switch to bottlefeeding. Even a couple of weeks of breastfeeding gets your baby off to a good start in life. It is more important that your baby gains the necessary weight than that you struggle along with a feeding method that isn't really working.

Before abandoning breastfeeding, consult a breastfeeding support group, such as La Lèche League (see the Useful addresses section at the back of the book for contact details), which has a publication specifically on breastfeeding your Down's syndrome baby. Getting support may be enough to help you through this difficult patch.

If you plan to combine breast- and bottlefeeding, it is worth mentioning that once babies have experienced a bottle and find it easier going than the breast, they may well not be so keen on the work that breastfeeding involves!

Weaning

The weaning process is much the same as with other babies – a gradual introduction of solids to back up milk feeds. However, see the advice given by the Down's Clinic in London (at www.jamont.freeserve.co.uk/lejeune), which, among other matters, recommends introducing iron-rich foods into the diet by six months to counteract the danger of iron deficiency. You will recall that earlier it was noted that children with Down's syndrome can be more prone to this than other children. Also aim to include foods rich in folic acid and antioxidant vitamins and minerals (for more on diet, see Chapter 9).

While you should encourage your child to be independent in feeding and master finger foods even if a spoon is too difficult, you may also need to ask your doctor, dentist or other professional about any dietary alterations you need to make if your child does not yet have enough teeth to chew some foods (see also under 'Teething' below).

Other care

New babies are not very good at keeping themselves warm or cool enough as their temperature-regulating mechanism is immature at birth. This may be especially true of a baby with Down's syndrome. So, aim to keep your new baby warm but not hot, in a room at a temperature of at least 18°C, with no draughts. Cooled boiled water, offered regularly, can help prevent dehydration.

If your baby becomes cold, the quickest way to warm him or her is skin-to-skin contact. You could do this, for example, by holding your baby to you wrapped in a warm blanket (though be careful he or she doesn't then become too warm). As many babies with Down's syndrome breathe through their mouths and can have blocked up noses, it may help to keep the baby's room humidified.

Babies with Down's syndrome often have dry skin, so it can help to massage your baby with baby oil or E45 cream or put oil in the bath. If the skin is very dry, try putting Oilatum Bath Emollient in the bath. Watch for dryness, cracking or allergic-type reactions and consult your doctor if they occur.

Teething

Some studies suggest that children with Down's syndrome teethe later than other babies. The first teeth may arrive before your baby is one or as late as two. The last of the baby teeth may not come in until the age of five! If no teeth appear by 16 to 17 months, ask your dentist to check your baby's tooth development.

Children with Down's syndrome may have other dental concerns. Smaller than average jaws and dental arch may lead to problems with the way in which the upper and lower teeth are positioned – called *malocclusion*. Later, some teenagers will need braces and possibly to have one or more teeth removed as well.

The teeth tend to be generally smaller and may have more irregularities in shape than usual. There may be white or brown spots on the teeth from a deficiency in enamel.

On the positive side, there is some evidence that children with Down's syndrome have less tooth decay, though gum (periodontal) disease can occur, due to a poor immune system.

Good oral hygiene is very important, even before any teeth appear. Clean your baby's gums by wiping them with a cloth at least once a day. When the teeth appear, you can begin to brush them with a baby toothbrush and a dot of fluoride toothpaste. It is a good idea to take your baby to the dentist for an examination at this point and regularly from then on.

Many parents report that their children are acutely sensitive about the mouth, making tooth and mouth hygiene difficult. Some speech and language therapists (see Chapter 8) suggest gentle mouth massage to help desensitize the mouth. You may need to build up to this gradually by, for example, starting by massaging at the shoulders or even the trunk and then moving gradually up to the mouth.

Some children with Down's syndrome have a habit of grinding their teeth – known as bruxism. Most of the time, no treatment is needed, although some children may need a plastic bite guard. One little boy actually wore his teeth down to the nerves by constant grinding, so it can be a problem. Sometimes bruxism may be caused by chronic ear infections or be a response to chronic allergic conditions. As with other things, don't accept it as an inevitable part of Down's syndrome – check it out with your dentist and/or doctor.

Activities, toys and equipment

All babies benefit from 'stimulus' – that is, loving attention and play at the right time, which helps along emotional, mental and physical development. Many parents with Down's syndrome babies have reported how important this kind of activity is for a child who, in the words of one mother, may be more 'laid back' than others!

Stimulus doesn't have to be non-stop. Your baby needs time alone and quieter times, too. Babies show that they have switched off in different ways – yawning, blinking, sneezing, turning their heads away, staring into space or just going to sleep! Some babies with heart defects or other medical conditions may be too unwell for much stimulation at first. Watch your baby's reactions and keep stimulus brief and gentle if need be.

The following ideas are by no means exhaustive – you know your own baby best and once you start on the stimulation process, you will find out just what your baby likes and develop from there. Some items mentioned below may be helpful to mention as possible gifts to friends and family who want to buy something for the new baby but aren't sure what to get.

In the early days, your baby will probably enjoy hugs and cuddles and hearing you speak or sing to him or her. Try making a tape of you and your partner talking or crooning or of natural sounds or else play some classical music, such as Mozart and Bach (the so-called 'Mozart effect' does exist – classical music has been shown to stimulate the brain).

Your baby's vision is also developing and he or she may enjoy looking at black and white shapes or mobiles or a toy torch that has coloured lights, such as red and green. You can also help your baby develop visual tracking skills by slowly moving a toy to and fro before his or her eyes or bringing it close and then moving it back a little way. Your baby may also enjoy games that involve pulling faces, while a game of poking the tongue in and out may help tongue control.

Scents to smell is another idea, such as perfumed soap or a bag of spices.

As your baby's back control develops and he or she begins to kick, helping along body and spatial awareness is important so that he or she knows where his or her body ends and the rest of the world begins. Massage is one way of doing this (see below). Other ways are to place him or her, naked some of the time, on to different textures, such as a blanket, eiderdown, rug or even paper, such as baking paper. Swinging your baby on a blanket is another idea (with another adult taking the blanket's other end). Certain toys may encourage your baby to use his or her hands and legs, such as activity gyms and kicking keyboards, which can be placed at the end of a cot as well as above or at the side of a baby. Different toys, paper, bells or other objects can also be placed at the end of the cot for your baby to kick against. Likewise, a mobile can be made with household or natural objects – pieces of wood, spoons, balloons, a mirror.

The Down's Syndrome Association in the UK suggests giving your baby a bath with a big rolled-up towel laid in it, then placing the baby tummy down on top of the towel. In this position, an older baby may make crawling movements. For a younger baby, who will need to be gently supported in the water and placed tummy up, the rolled-up towel provides a new, interesting sensation.

As your baby's back control develops further, he or she may enjoy being in a bouncing chair to watch what is going on around the house. This is also a good way to give any extra body support that may be needed due to low muscle tone. Later, a stable, supportive highchair may also be helpful as it can prop up a baby who can't quite sit up. It comes in very useful for feeding when starting solids and also makes it easier for your baby to hold his or her own bottle or cup, manage finger foods or play with a toy once the manual dexterity needed to do so has developed.

Your baby will probably also enjoy all the traditional baby toys, such as rattles or any toys that make a sound or light up when shaken, stimulating curiosity as well as hand control. Once your baby is more mobile – perhaps rolling, reaching or thinking about crawling – you can encourage him or her to move by placing a toy just out of reach. A touch of frustration spurs many babies on in their development!

Contact and massage

Your baby will probably love a gentle massage – perhaps sometimes on just one part of the body, such as the fingers or feet. He or she may also love being carried in a sling, skin to skin if possible. Other ideas for gentle physical stimulus include blowing or tickling or tapping the face and body gently with your fingertips.

Miriam Kauk, mother of Mary, 8, runs a comprehensive website on Down's syndrome (www.einstein-syndrome.com) and suggests facial massage in order to tone up muscle tones and avoid any slackness:

As your baby learns to control some of her facial muscles, necessary for smiling and speech, begin to gently massage her entire face, around the mouth, eyes, forehead, cheeks, temples, and even the back of her head. Do one minute lightly, then a minute firmly tap-tapping.

This technique was originally recommended by Bob Doman, founder of the National Academy for Child Development, Utah, USA, who has evolved several neurodevelopmental programmes for children with learning disabilities.

71

Responsive babies

Most babies with Down's syndrome are warm and cuddly, hugely enjoy contact with their parents and show the smallest delay of all in their social and emotional development. Paul Rogers and Mary Coleman, authors of the book *Medical Care in Down Syndrome: A Preventive Medicine Approach* (1992), say that you can expect a baby with Down's syndrome to:

- smile when talked to at 2 months (range 1.5–4 months)
- smile spontaneously at 3 months (range 2–6 months)
- recognize parents at 3.5 months (range 3–6 months).

Each milestone shows only around a month delay on average. Babies with Down's syndrome begin to enjoy pat-a-cake and peek-a-boo games at about 11 months (range 9–16 months), which is about 3 months later than other babies.

Studies carried out in Down's babies' second year show that they are skilled social communicators, even using certain skills to try and distract an adult from a task the baby didn't want to attempt! Research also shows that this normal emotional responsiveness develops into empathy and social awareness.

8

What to expect as your child grows up

The early years are a time of great development, seeing the emergence of not just skills but also your child's personality and a growing relationship with you and with others. Children with Down's syndrome do particularly well in a loving, supportive environment. It may be a myth that they are invariably happy and affectionate – many mothers testify to a normal level of parental irritation caused by a lively, sometimes bolshy child who enjoys having his or her own way! However, it is true that consistent support from you can bring out the best in your child, helping to develop to his or her full potential.

Perhaps the most vital emerging issue in the first few years is motor development – how your child learns to move around. While there are broadly three main areas of development – motor, cognitive and social – motor development tends to be the first great marker of how your child is doing, what his or her capabilities are, how he or she learns, solves problems and copes with frustrations. Mobility is also vital to your child's overall development because babies learn by moving around and exploring their environment. The ability to sit up and look around, grasp a mobile or crawl to a cupboard, open it and pull out objects – all are motor skills that encourage understanding of the environment, so stimulating cognitive, language and social development.

Communication and speech form another key area. In the years before a child can read and write (though some children with Down's syndrome can read at age three – see the next chapter!), how he or she communicates with those around him or her is a touchstone of personality, social skills and understanding. There are, of course, numerous other issues, such as behaviour, nutrition and starting playgroup, nursery and school, which are also covered in the next chapter.

While this chapter looks primarily at skills that are likely to start emerging in the toddler years, which are around the ages of one to three or four, the importance of early intervention (described below) means that it can be very helpful to look at these issues while your child is still a baby. Many parents feel that it has proved vital that they started therapy, such as physical and speech therapy, in infancy.

One suggestion. Most children will make steady developmental progress, so many parents find it satisfying to collect together and celebrate these little and great triumphs, not just in the red book used in the UK to record the results of developmental checks, but in a personalized book of photos, thoughts and memories.

Your child's development

Your child will learn skills such as holding her head steady, sitting, crawling and standing, though they may all be learned some months later than usual.

All children develop according to individual timetables anyway, but this is even truer of those with Down's syndrome. For example, according to Cliff Cunningham, Professor of Applied Psychology at Liverpool John Moores University and author of *Understanding Down Syndrome: An Introduction for Parents* (1996), your child with Down's syndrome may sit alone at 6 to 16 months rather than 5 to 9 months as in typical development and walk at 1 to 4 years, rather than 9 to 17 months (these are termed gross motor skills); he or she may build a tower of two blocks at 14 to 32 months, as opposed to the usual 10 to 19 months (these are fine motor skills); he or she may say a first word at 1 to 3 years, instead of 10 to 23 months; he or she may start to eat finger foods at 6 to 14 months, rather than 4 to 10 months (social development); and be toilet trained by 2 to 7 years rather than 1 to 3 years.

As you can see, there is huge variation in the ages at which individual children may develop different skills. Sometimes illness may slow a child down. Generally, though, it is probably more helpful to look at the sequence of milestones achieved, rather than the ages at which they were reached. This is because development is rather like building blocks – the first block needs to be in place before the others can be added. In motor development, for example, while most parents eagerly look for the day when their baby first walks, learning to hold the head steady is the first of many developmental steps that eventually lead to walking. This is because motor development proceeds according to the *cephalocaudal law*, which is that development starts from the head and proceeds downwards. This is why a child learns to control the head first and walk later. Motor development also proceeds according to the *proximodistal law*. This means that development proceeds from the centre outwards, which explains why hand control comes relatively later on in the developmental process.

According to Patricia Winders, physical therapist and author of *Gross Motor Skills in Children with Down Syndrome: A Guide for Parents and Professionals* (1997), the rate of motor development in children with Down's syndrome is influenced by four factors: lack of muscle control, slacker ligaments than usual (they hold the bones together), leading to increased flexibility in the joints, less muscle strength and short arms and legs relative to the size of the trunk. All these are laid down by genetics and cannot be changed by therapy.

Early intervention

Even taking into account all the above, most professionals stress the importance of early intervention for a child with Down's syndrome. Essentially, this means early help with aspects of development so that your child will achieve his or her maximum potential without being pushed.

Early intervention programmes provided by local health authorities vary but may include physiotherapy, speech and language therapy and occupational therapy. It's generally recommended that the earlier intervention is started, the better, but consult the professionals involved in your child's care for guidance.

Some programmes of education or therapy may be designed to speed up the development of preschool children with disabilities. However, it may be more helpful to look on early intervention as encouraging skills to emerge according to the individual child's timetable.

Motor skills, more than other developmental skills, depend on brain maturity and so a child cannot be taught, say, to sit and walk before he or she is physically ready. However, early intervention may help counteract the tendency to poor muscle tone and so, once ready, your child will be able to benefit more from opportunities to practise new skills.

Some studies have found that physical therapy does seem to help children acquire motor skills earlier, but this needs to be balanced by the child's long-term needs. For example, children with Down's syndrome may find walking more difficult than other children because they tend to have decreased muscle tone and strength, more flexible joints and shorter arms and legs than them.

According to American research, children with Down's syndrome can learn to walk earlier and better by regularly exercising on a slow treadmill as this helps them develop the necessary leg strength and posture control. A study at the University of Michigan's Center for Motor Behavior in Down Syndrome found that children who used a treadmill regularly started walking three and a half months sooner than those who did not receive the therapy. The children practised on a slow treadmill with a parent for just eight minutes a day, five days a week.

Another small study at Liverpool John Moores University in the UK found that formal training led to significant improvement in children with Down's syndrome acquiring running skills, which on average appear two years later than in typical development.

Any early intervention and physical therapy needs to keep the child's long-term motor skills in mind, not just short-term reaching of milestones. While the age at which a baby walks is one of the first key milestones for parents, it is better that your child learns to walk at his or her own pace, with the supervision of a therapist if necessary, than that he or she learns to walk early.

Physical therapy may not speed up the rate of motor development, but it could help to prevent your child from adopting abnormal compensatory movement patterns, such as poor posture, standing with the tummy pushed out and back arched, walking with the feet wide apart – an inefficient and often painful way to get around – or abnormal spine curvature due to low muscle tone in the trunk, which in turn results in poor head posture and breathing patterns.

Cognitive and social development can also be addressed by early intervention in the form of general education intervention programmes. The Portage Home Teaching Scheme, for example, provides activities to help progress motor skills, language, independence and understanding (see the Useful addresses section at the back of the book for contact details).

Any early intervention should begin with a thorough assessment of a baby's health to ensure that this will not interfere with his or her development.

How children with Down's syndrome learn

Research suggests that children with Down's syndrome have a different learning style from that which is typical for children of their age.

- They may have less ability to generalize and will probably process information better if it is in small, bite-sized pieces.
- New information and skills need to be introduced slowly and carefully, allowing time and repeating things as necessary to help them gradually absorb information.
- They also need structure, consistency and a familiar environment.
- Ideally, they learn best when you follow their lead.
- It helps to keep frustration to a minimum and give them plenty of experiences of success.
- Like other children, they may be good at wriggling out of tasks they dislike! Gentle encouragement to stay with it may be needed.
- They tend to be visual learners – that is, they process sights more easily than sounds, whether as a result of hearing problems or other reasons.
- They may also have poor memories and forget what they've been told, whether it is the name of a book or when to go to lunch.

You will have plenty of chances to assess your own child's particular learning style, but one of the earliest opportunities is at the point when he or she starts to use motor skills. How your child handles these challenges will give vital clues about his or her general learning style. For example, would your child charge into a shopping bag the minute you put it down or be slow and careful about approaching new situations?

Exercise

Because of a certain lack of muscle tone and developmental delays, some children will take longer than others to learn skills such as running, jumping, skipping, throwing and catching. However, there is no reason for your child not to enjoy some kind of physical activity, adapting what you do to suit his or her individual level of ability. As well as boosting general fitness, exercise can lessen the likelihood of obesity. One study found that children with Down's syndrome were likely to take part in less physical activity than other children, suggesting that the greater levels of obesity may be due to lack of activity rather than Down's syndrome itself. Although some studies have found that people with Down's syndrome do not benefit as much from exercise as people without Down's syndrome, other researchers have concluded that those who become physically active do improve their strength and endurance. Exercise has also been suggested as a measure to improve blood flow to the brain, so potentially protecting against Alzheimer's disease, which people with Down's syndrome have a high risk of developing at a young age. However, this has not yet been tested.

Fitness has social as well as health benefits. The fitter your child, the greater the opportunities for joining in play and sport with other children, reducing the frustration and anxiety felt at not being able to join in.

Some children with Down's syndrome will need to take more care with exercise than others. Children with heart problems may lack stamina and so need to take little breaks from time to time in order to rest. Some children may have poor circulation, which may cause them to either overheat or become very cold. What kind of exercise is suitable for your child and how much is something that you should check with your doctor.

Other difficulties include neck instability or orthopaedic problems, such as dislocating hips and knees or flat feet, respiratory problems and chest infections, as well as, more rarely, seizures. Consult your doctor before starting an exercise programme if you have any doubts about whether or not your child's health allows him or her to exercise safely.

Once given the medical all-clear, there is no reason for your child not to join a sports or exercise class, though you may need to explain your child's level of ability to the teacher.

Some children with Down's syndrome may need a little extra encouragement to get going. Annabel speaks of the 'pushchair syndrome' – mothers continuing to wheel round older toddlers perfectly capable of walking just because it's safer and they know where the child is. However, this does not contribute to the child's physical well-being! In fitness as in other areas of life, expectations can be key. They need to be high, but realistic! Annabel points out that children who have everything done for them are unlikely to learn independence: 'Some children I know can't put their coats on at age 10 – but I strongly suspect that this is because a parent has always been there to put the coat on for them!'

Communication and speech

More than 95 per cent of children with Down's syndrome will use speech as their primary communication system. However, as with motor skills, 'speech' starts well before the first word is spoken and is built on a process that includes cooing, babbling and making and imitating sounds. Babies communicate in many other ways before using speech itself – facial expressions, smiles, gestures and sounds. In typical development, these preverbal exchanges usually pose no problems to the parents and child communicating. Games with you also help build the basis for future conversational skills. For example, peek-a-boo games are a way of developing turn-taking. The most important foundation for these games is your baby's social awareness, which is not usually a problem for children with Down's syndrome.

To learn to speak, your child also needs other skills, such as listening skills, cognitive skills (such as understanding object permanence – that objects continue to exist even when not in sight) and tactile skills (learning about touch, exploring objects in the mouth and so on, which may present difficulties if your child is subject to oral hypersensitivity). Also needed are good mouth and tongue muscle control – an area where children with Down's syndrome may have difficulty. Your child may have trouble forming words because of the smaller than usual mouth cavity that is part of the syndrome.

While the speech and language problems faced by children with Down's syndrome are experienced by other children as well, some are more likely than others. Many children with Down's syndrome find understanding what is said (receptive language) much easier than talking themselves (expressive language). This happens typically in all children's development as understanding speech is always ahead of speech itself, but the difficulty may persist longer in a child with Down's syndrome.

Other areas, such as vocabulary, may in fact be easier for children with Down's syndrome than other children, while more difficult areas may be grammar, the sequencing of sounds and words, fluency and intelligibility of speech and articulation.

Some children also have difficulties processing speech in their minds that affect their perception of words. They may also have limitations in their auditory short-term memory – that is, they quickly forget what they have been told because they have trouble storing and processing units of information relating to, for example, words and their meanings or instructions.

All this means that patience and time will be needed before your child is able to use words to communicate. Frustratingly for them, many children with Down's syndrome can understand the relationship between a word and a concept by around one year old, but not yet have the necessary neurological and motor skills to be able to speak.

One way round this is to use an interim means of communication, such as signing, which children with Down's syndrome often take to readily because it is visual. Most children with Down's syndrome are ready to use a communication system many months or even years before they are able to use speech. Using signing systems is another way to help a child who wants to communicate but hasn't yet developed the physical mechanisms for making words. Some systems use signs and gestures in combination with speech to teach language. Some parents worry that their child will become dependent on this system, but it is designed as a transitional system and research shows that most children drop it once they can speak so as to make themselves understood.

Early speech therapy

Many parents and experts believe that there is a case for starting speech-directed therapy well before speech itself. This is because oral motor skills – such as moving the tongue and lips – are needed for speech, but, due to lack of muscle tone, this is an area where children with Down's syndrome have difficulties.

Breathing and feeding involve many of the structures and muscles later used in speech, and some forms of therapy directed at oral motor skills may help a child further to prepare for speech. Therapy can help strengthen the oral muscles used in feeding and speech alike, giving children practice with strengthening and coordinating the muscles that will be used for speech.

> I would like to share my feelings about the importance of speech therapy input from an age much earlier than might be imagined. It is vital not to wait until the child is ready to talk – and the role of a therapist would be to spot any early oral motor problems as well as to teach the parents or carers signing.
>
> I had a big issue with accepting signing, because it seemed like such an admission of disability, and wonder if it could have been better explained when Luke was very small. He has now hit the magical age of six, when I think something special happens and the speech itself kicks in, but it would have given him more contact with his immediate world if he had learnt Makaton signing and if we had used it as a family. Children with Down's are particularly visually inspired, so signing works very well for them. That is something I understood a little too late.
> *Jo, mother of Luke*

One particular feature of Down's syndrome is that, quite often, the children hate being touched, especially around the mouth. They may hate having their teeth brushed or dislike certain textures of foods.

Libby Kumin, Professor of Speech-language Pathology at Loyola College in Maryland, and Diane Chapman, a speech-language pathologist in Baltimore, Maryland, use a massage programme aimed at gradually overcoming the acute sensitivity to touching the mouth often found in children with Down's syndrome. As a result, this facilitates prespeech activity, such as babbling and making sounds. The massage programme begins with the arms and legs and gradually moves towards the face and mouth area. Research suggests that, in this way, babies and toddlers come increasingly to tolerate touch in the lip and tongue area and that they do more babbling and sound-making after such therapy than would otherwise be the case. Once the child can tolerate touch and freely move the parts of the mouth needed for speech, an oral motor skills programme is introduced. This might include blowing whistles, blowing bubbles, making funny faces and imitating sounds. All these things can be done easily at home with the guidance of a speech therapist.

Music therapy, such as singing, may also help a child to practise prespeech skills and oral control.

How to help with language development

Once your child is starting to speak, research on language development suggests that it is very helpful if you do the following.

- Most children with Down's syndrome learn words better after many repetitions and experiences of using them. Repeat what your child says and use games, activities and toys to help him or her learn words.
- Reading to your child helps with learning vocabulary and concepts.
- Listen to your child and take him or her seriously. Most children with Down's syndrome enjoy conversations if you follow their lead.
- Allow plenty of time for your child to muster his or her thoughts and get the words out. Don't be afraid of pauses or jump in with too many suggestions or requests.
- Finally, given that 60–80 per cent of young children with Down's syndrome may have a hearing problem at some time in childhood, it is worth repeating how important it is to get your child's hearing regularly checked so that any hearing loss can either be prevented or overcome, avoiding greater language and speech delay, as well as frustration being experienced by your child.

Remember, language is about far more than just the spoken word. What your child relishes is the full range of communication with you – cuddling, watching TV or reading a book together, singing or listening to music. There are many powerful communication tools and perhaps none makes a child feel more valued than the simple act of sitting down with him or her and giving of your time – time in which he or she can take as long as is needed to communicate what is important to him or her, in his or her own way, without distractions.

Communicating positively with your child is vital to helping him or her feel valued and confident, as well as being an important building block in good, nurturing relationships with others.

9

Daily life with your child

Although there is no cure for Down's syndrome, it is possible to prevent many of the problems associated with the condition and to ensure that your child reaches his or her full potential in terms of happiness, education and everyday interests. This chapter looks at ways in which to boost your child's health and well-being, including diet, toilet training, sleeping well and starting school.

Boosting general health

Given the vulnerable immunity system of the child with Down's syndrome, many parents try a variety of measures to boost health.

Jo arranged for Luke to have cranial osteopathy (also called craniosacral therapy) from two weeks old and he still enjoys a treatment session from time to time today. Jo has found this to be of immense benefit. She also saw an acupuncturist to cure a never-ending ear infection when Luke's doctor was ready to fit him with grommets.

Tiffany tried aromatherapy on Jacquie in babyhood, but, although she seemed to enjoy it, Tiffany found it too expensive to continue with. Instead, she massaged Jacquie herself, adding a drop of lavender oil to some baby oil. Jacquie seemed to relish this just as much as the sessions with the professional aromatherapist.

Diet

A healthy diet is of major importance for children with Down's syndrome as they tend not to grow as tall as other children, so can find that they put on weight easily. Do consult your doctor and health visitor for information about your child's particular needs, but, otherwise, the whole family can benefit from following a healthy eating plan that includes lots of fresh fruits and vegetables, avoids saturated fats and fried foods, and with cakes, sweets and other goodies saved for occasional treats. Ensure that your child has enough liquid, fibre and exercise to counteract constipation and be sure to contact your doctor if recurring tummy troubles are a worry (see Chapter 6).

Some parents have their children follow special diets as a way of improving their general health. These include specialized exclusion diets – for example, gluten-free for a child who has coeliac disease (see Chapter 6) – taking vitamin and mineral supplements and so on. This last is rather controversial. It has long been believed that certain food supplements might help improve the health of children with Down's syndrome, though there is currently no hard and fast scientific evidence for this. For example, Lejeune found that many children with Down's syndrome were lacking iron and folic acid, but later studies have disputed this. Other studies have suggested that the diets of children with Down's syndrome are more likely to be deficient in fibre, calcium, zinc and copper. The 1980s saw a great deal of research into megadoses of vitamins and minerals and their effect on the intelligence and mental functioning of those with Down's syndrome. Unfortunately, none of the studies showed them to have a definitive beneficial effect. More recent work has also looked at amino acids, with no conclusive results.

Research has suggested that children with Down's syndrome may not absorb enough nutrients from their diet because of defects in how they metabolize nutrients, including vitamins, minerals, anti-oxidants and amino acids. In addition, some children with Down's syndrome may also suffer from malabsorption, coeliac disease and lactose intolerance (see Chapter 6).

It's also been suggested that children with Down's syndrome may be more vulnerable to free radical damage than other children and so need more antioxidants such as vitamin C, betacarotene, vitamin E and selenium. In the body, oxygen can be converted into free radicals, which can cause tissue damage and possibly accelerate the ageing process and degeneration of the brain, and perhaps, therefore, contribute towards the health problems associated with Down's syndrome, such as short stature, developmental difficulties, increased likelihood of infections and later susceptibility to developing Alzheimer's-type dementia.

An example of a nutritional therapy based on such thinking is Targeted Nutritional Intervention (TNI). It makes use of a compli-cated blend of vitamins, minerals, amino acids and digestive enzymes. TNI is designed to reverse or at least lessen some of the effects of Down's syndrome, such as long-term degeneration, though it is not promoted as a cure or panacea for unhealthy eating habits. Supplements are not meant to replace a healthy diet but to do as their name suggests and support and boost such a diet.

Such nutritional programmes, though reported to be helpful by some individuals, have not been subjected to clinical trials. In particular, concerns have been expressed that some of them make use of medicines (such as piracetam) that are not licensed for use in children with Down's syndrome. In addition, the suggested doses for the nutritional supplements are often much higher than the recommended maximum safe doses. In the end, the only kind of proof for them is anecdotal – that is, reports from other parents who have tried these approaches.

Jo tried Luke on TNI – excluding any medicines, and focusing instead just on the supplements of vitamins and minerals. Luke had just three colds in his life until he started playgroup, when, in the normal way, he began picking up germs from other children. Jo discontinued TNI largely because of the expense – not only were the supplements costly at that time, but also they were only available from the USA and so she had to pay huge amounts of duty on them, despite wrangles with the customs authorities as to the supposed duty-free status of therapeutic supplies for children with disabilities. (TNI can now be bought in the UK – see the Useful addresses section at the back of the book for contact details.)

Warning: **Consult your doctor before starting your child on any nutritional programme.**

Most people tend to get sufficient omega 6 fats from their diet via nuts, seeds and oils. However, many of us do not eat enough oily fish (we should be eating one to two servings a week). Do also bear in mind that nuts and seeds carry a danger of choking for small children and some are allergic to them, so be cautious – perhaps serving them well-ground in biscuits made with minimal amounts of sugar.

Antioxidants, omega 3 and omega 6

The Down's Syndrome Research Foundation (DSRF) – a body that aims to encourage more research into Down's syndrome – believes that the main value of programmes such as TNI is due to the antioxidants they contain. So, could antioxidant vitamins and minerals help children with Down's syndrome?

Doctors at the Institutes of Child Health in London and Birmingham are trying to find out the answer to this question, together with the Jérôme Lejeune Foundation in Paris and the Down's Syndrome Research Foundation, which provided initial funding for this project. The study, the biggest of its kind, is looking at vitamins A, C, E, zinc and selenium and folinic acid – a form of folic acid. Information on the study is available at the website: www.cddg-downs.org.uk

Meanwhile, the DSRF's initial findings suggest that, in addition, omega 3 and omega 6 oils are valuable. These are available as supplements at healthfood shops, but are best taken as part of a healthy diet. Taking enough supplements such as these may, the DSRF suggests, increase brain growth and reduce cell damage. At any rate, a healthy diet consisting of foods rich in these nutrients can only be good for your child's general health.

- *Antioxidants* are found in fresh fruit and vegetables.
- *Omega 3* is found in fish, especially oily fish such as mackerel, lake trout, herring, sardines, pilchards, fresh tuna, salmon and cod liver oil – all of which contain a form of omega 3, docosahexaenoic acid (DHA), essential for brain growth. Another form of omega 3, alpha-linolenic acid (ALA), can be found in flax seed (linseed) oil, rapeseed (canola) oil, chia seeds, walnuts and walnut oil, tofu and other forms of soya beans, green leafy vegetables, grains and spirulina.
- *Omega 6* is found in vegetable seeds and polyunsaturated margarine, safflower, sunflower, corn, soya or evening primrose oils and wheatgerm.

Toilet training

Successful toilet training in all children depends on the maturing of the nervous system and this tends to develop later in children with Down's syndrome, as do their powers of coordination. It is unrealistic to start thinking about training until your child is over the age of three, though this, too, will depend on your individual child and his or her temperament.

The best time to start is when you feel that your child is aware that he or she has wet or soiled a nappy. Once your child does know this, try sitting him or her on a potty, if possible at a time when you know that something may be produced. If something is, give lots of praise. Once he or she can tell you in advance when to get the potty, try trainer pants. Again, give lots of praise when your child succeeds.

Choose to start at a time when you are relaxed and there are not going to be too many interruptions. It is a good idea to try in the summer so you can be outside, if possible. When you move on to using the toilet, many children like a little step to help them to climb up and also appreciate a smaller, slip-on seat.

Sleep problems

There is some evidence that children with Down's syndrome can be more prone to sleep problems than other children. According to sleep expert Dr Rebecca Stores of the University of Oxford, some 50 per cent of children with Down's syndrome may have problems, among the most common of which are difficulties settling children to sleep and waking during the night. Persistent sleep disturbance can cause a number of problems in your child, including behaviour problems, irritability, hyperactivity, aggression, learning problems and reduced attention and concentration. Lack of sleep may also worsen any areas of delay in your child, including growth delay (especially if your child has sleep apnoea – growth hormone is only released during deep sleep). Such problems may be misinterpreted as being 'just part of Down's syndrome', but you shouldn't accept this.

Interrupted sleep causes a huge strain for the rest of the family, leading to stress and irritability. Perhaps most importantly, though, interrupted sleep in your child can be a symptom of a sleep-related disorder that needs specialist medical attention – particularly obstructive sleep apnoea syndrome (see Chapter 6, Health issues, under the heading 'Sleep apnoea'). Therefore, before starting any sleep training with your child, it is important to see your doctor first. Apart from the possibility of sleep-related breathing disorders, you also need to exclude any illness that could be interrupting sleep, such as an ear infection. Usually, though, it is a matter of needing to teach your child to sleep without you – something he or she may never have learned.

Sleep medications are not usually advised (because they don't work in the long term) unless they are advised as a very short-term measure to help you through a crisis. Research indicates that long-term sleep training works much better and is much better for your child. Here's how you can help your child.

- Set a bedtime routine – for example, by including regular events such as the evening meal, wind-down time, bath. Keep it simple. If you don't have a clear routine, it may take your child several weeks to get used to having one, but it is worth persevering.
- Let your child make some bedtime choices, such as what to wear or what book to read.
- Anticipate any requests – story, cuddle, drink – and make them part of your bedtime routine. Allow one extra request, but make it clear that one is the limit.
- Try keeping a sleep diary for two weeks. Record not only how many hours of sleep your child is getting, but also other possible influences on sleep, such as diet, including stimulants such as sugar and food additives, exercise or any activities that seem to upset your child.
- Exercise is certainly useful in ensuring that your child is tired enough to sleep, but shouldn't occur too close to bedtime in case it is overstimulating (this applies to everyone, of course). Mid-afternoon may be a good time – perhaps just after school if it can be managed.
- Helping your child to wind down before bedtime is important, as it is for all children and, indeed, adults! It can give you a chance to relax, too.
- Cut out daytime naps if you think that they are interfering with sleep. You may need to do this gradually.
- Ensure that the room is cosy, warm and quiet enough, using nightlights, cuddly toys and comforters, if your child likes them. In summer, make sure that the curtains are heavy enough to exclude light. If not, you can get blackout curtain linings.

- Once you have said goodnight, don't give in to any more demands for drinks, stories and so on.
- If your child wakes during the night, try to avoid taking him or her into your bed.
- Praise and reward your child when he or she does sleep well.

If you like, you can train your child using the checking method. This involves returning at regular intervals to ensure that your child is all right while staying calm and kind, but firm. Soothe your child briefly, then leave. Go in at ever-increasing intervals – that is, first leave your child for one minute, then two, then five. Ideally, your child knows that you are around, but should get the message that it is night and time to sleep. This method has been criticized as being too harsh, but it can work very well for some hardened offenders, given a few nights.

A gentler approach is the gradual withdrawal method. You say goodnight at ever further distances from the bed – for example, from the bedroom door or hall, rather than going in.

Both methods can be very hard to keep to if your child cries, especially in the middle of the night, but they can work if you allow at least three nights. If you are going to give in, it's probably best to do so at once, otherwise you teach your child that persistence can and does wear you down. You can always try again when you feel stronger or try a different approach. If you need support – and sticking with it can be very hard – ask your doctor if any sleep clinics are available to help.

Behaviour

As with other aspects of Down's syndrome, there are several myths surrounding the supposed personality of those with Down's syndrome – placid, obstinate, sluggish and so on. Behaviour problems may be related to any of a number of accompanying problems, such as poor health, not Down's syndrome itself. Sometimes a child will communicate by means of anger and frustration if he or she doesn't have the language to explain the feelings being experienced. Other factors include boredom, lack of understanding or the child's immature development. Jo found that Luke was displaying aggressive behaviour and having tantrums at school. She couldn't understand this as Luke usually loved the other children, but then she realized that, at six, he was showing behaviour appropriate to the toddler years: 'I hadn't realized that the delayed development would manifest itself in different ways, and that this was one way. Luke was going through a normal phase, but at an older age.'

Set limits and make sure that your child adheres to them in the same way as any other child. Clear boundaries and a predictable routine can help your child to learn what is expected and allay any anxiety about change. House rules, such as sitting still at meals, can help teach basic disciplinary skills that will make your child's life easier later at school, as can daily duties, such as brushing teeth or dressing. Do acknowledge any success, however small, with praise.

Keeping any commands short and clear ensures that there is no possibility of misunderstanding. Some children are quite skilled at using avoidance techniques when faced with a task that they dislike!

Do check so that you can exclude the possibility of illness causing bad behaviour – for example, pain from an ear infection. Also, ensure that any tasks do lie within your child's capabilities or else frustration will be caused.

The time-honoured strategy of rewarding good behaviour and ignoring the bad, if possible, can be effective. Be clear that it is the behaviour you are focusing on, not the child. So, say 'Throwing things is wrong' rather than 'You're a naughty boy to throw things.' Avoid unwittingly encouraging bad behaviour, such as shouting at your child. This only gives your child negative attention, which can, perversely, be a reward.

Starting playgroup

Preschools offer lots of opportunities for children to learn through play. Most offer a government-approved early years curriculum. Playgroups give your child a valuable taste of social life, offering a safe and stimulating environment in which to make friends and learn what it is like to form part of a group. Usually, too, you will be welcome to stay with your child as parental involvement is often a vital part of a playgroup.

Your child is entitled to a place at playgroup and you may wish to discuss this with your health visitor. You can also try ChildcareLink, which is a government service that provides information and advice on childcare (freephone 0800 096 0296; website: www.childcarelink. gov.uk). Try your local authority, too, or the Preschool Learning Alliance (020 7833 0991) for possible contacts.

It is best to visit several playgroups and talk to the playgroup leader about your child and any special needs. It may also be helpful to talk to other parents about which are the best playgroups in the area.

The Local Education Authority (LEA) may be able to help your child from a very early age. If your child is under two, you can ask the LEA to assess his or her needs. If your child is over two, you can ask the LEA to make a Statutory Assessment (see Getting your child statemented, below).

Getting your child statemented

It may be helpful to organize this by the time your child starts school or nursery. If it is drawn up too early, the information in it may be out of date by the time your child starts school, as these are years when major developmental changes occur. It's generally recommended, therefore, that you get the assessment process started around a year before the statement needs to be ready.

The assessment process itself takes at least 26 weeks, while an appeal, if necessary, takes 4 to 5 months. Getting a Statement is achieved in one of two main ways by your LEA. The LEA may contact you directly if it has information about your child from your local health authority. Alternatively, you can write to the Director of Education at your LEA, stating that your child has Down's syndrome, and request a full formal assessment of your child's special educational needs under section 323 of the Education Act 1996. For more information, see a booklet written by Sally Capper, Education Advocacy Worker for the Down's Syndrome Association UK, entitled 'A Guide to the Statement of Special Educational Needs' (see the Useful addresses section at the back of the book for contact details).

Making the transition to school

It is likely that your child will attend an ordinary primary school. There are around 16,000 school-age children with Down's syndrome

– it is the most common single cause of learning disabilities. Increasingly, it is expected that these children will attend mainstream schools and, indeed, children with Down's syndrome are quite capable of going to school and learning. Most will need a Statement of Special Educational Needs so that any extra resources they require can be provided (see Getting your child statemented, above).

Increasingly, children included at primary school will remain with their classmates and move on to a mainstream secondary school. Very many children with Down's syndrome are 'educable'. This word was formerly used as a kind of judgement of the cut-off point when deciding whether or not people should be confined within an institution and it used to be believed that children with Down's syndrome were maybe 'trainable' but not 'educable'. Today, the pendulum has swung and the emphasis is on inclusion as far as possible. Because of treatment in the past, we have yet to discover the full educational potential of people with Down's syndrome.

Some schools may be anxious about accepting children with Down's syndrome and dealing with the wide variety of needs they may present teachers with. However, in the UK, the Down's Syndrome Association has an Education Support Pack for Schools and this can be downloaded from its website (www.downs-syndrome.org.uk). It may also help to discuss issues with teachers directly (see What to discuss with your child's teacher, below).

Academic research has shown that children with disabilities perform better when included in an ordinary class, though cynics say that inclusion is championed merely because it is cheaper than the provision of exclusively special needs education. However, going to mainstream school gives children with Down's syndrome the chance to mix with other children from their own area and have a place in the local community. Mainstream schools provide good peer role models – shown to be helpful for children with Down's syndrome. Equally, it gives other children the chance to learn about children with special needs, which can be a foundation for social tolerance. While most children with Down's syndrome will be allocated extra support, such as a learning support assistant (LSA), it is important for your child's independence and growth that he or she is accepted as part of the class, not exclusively doing one-to-one work off to one side. Sometimes trouble is caused if a child feels excluded from exciting activities that the rest of the class is undertaking.

Learning to read

Until quite recently, it was thought that only an exceptional child with Down's syndrome would be able to read. However, research has shown that children with Down's syndrome as young as three years of age are succeeding at reading single words.

In the UK, Sue Buckley, at the University of Portsmouth, has done a lot of pioneering work in this area. She has found that, among other things, reading enhances speech in children with Down's syndrome and that they often find learning to read both easy and fun. (For more details on Sue Buckley's work, visit: www.down-syndrome.net) It is now recognized that reading and writing are all interrelated as language and communication skills.

Here are some tips for helping your child to prepare for reading:

- read as much as possible – at bedtime, in the bath, in the car – using a variety of books both with and without words
- share reading – let your child point to pictures or act out what is going on in the story and talk about the characters and plot
- make your own books with photos and your child's drawings and scribbles.

What to discuss with your child's teacher

(See also How children with Down's syndrome learn, in Chapter 8.)

While your child's teacher may be educated about Down's syndrome, it may still be helpful to have a few points for discussion if needed. Good communication with the school is vital to ensure that there is continuity between what happens at school and what happens at home.

It's important to recognize that Down's syndrome is not just another learning difficulty, but has a 'specific profile' of which teachers should be aware. At the same time, it's also vital to recognize that each child is an individual with his or her own temperament and that it may not be relevant to blame aspects of behaviour on Down's syndrome. In the interests of inclusion, it is probably wise not to make too much of your child's 'disability', but, rather, just give a few key facts to help ensure a smooth transition to school. Here are some suggestions for the kinds of point that it would be helpful to make.

- Children with Down's syndrome are primarily visual learners – they learn best by seeing and doing. For example, reading may need to be taught by sight rather than sound, often by recognizing the shapes of whole words, not phonics.
- They often have poor short-term memories and forget what they've been told, whether it's the name of a book or when to go to lunch. The teacher may therefore need to repeat class instructions on a one-to-one basis.
- Due to language delay, they may still use short phrases when other children are forming full sentences. They may also need more time than average to respond to questions. Specific language difficulties, such as problems understanding or retaining instructions and difficulty speaking intelligibly, may also need to be mentioned.
- They may have a short concentration span and work best if activities are kept short and focused.
- They may have problems with physical coordination, leading to clumsiness, and not be very good at PE. However, if their health permits, it is important that they join in without being overprotected.
- Children with any sight or hearing problems obviously need to be placed at the front of the class. The teacher may need to repeat what is being said, perhaps using gestures and visual aids as well.
- Many children with Down's syndrome dislike changes to a routine so may need more time to adjust to any new moves, such as having lunch outside in the summer rather than inside as normal.

Building a good school–home relationship can take time, but is definitely worth it in terms of peace of mind. One of the quickest and easiest ways to get to know a school is to offer to help with reading or other classroom activities – most schools are only too pleased to accept parent volunteer help, whether this is just for an hour or so occasionally or more. Some schools, as a matter of policy, prefer not to have parents help in their own child's class, but at least by going in you can get a feel for the school, as well as improve communication with those responsible for your child's care.

10

Other issues

After the initial shock, families often begin to adapt and feel more positive and optimistic, showing great determination to create the best possible quality of life for their child with Down's syndrome. Getting to know their baby usually does away with all those grim fears of the unknown that contribute so much to the initial shock factor. So does watching their child develop into a toddler, at their own pace and seeing their life expand.

This process usually involves adjusting expectations and values.

> I found it hard to change my expectations of what constitutes success, both for me and my child. Am I a successful mother if I produce a 'genetically flawed' child? Is Jack not a success if he isn't toilet trained and only has a few words at three? I found I had to replace a concept of success through attainment ('doing' things) with a concept of less tangible achievements – a whole different way of thinking and being. There are times when I still find it hard and get frustrated now because our whole culture is against this way of thinking, even if it pays lip-service to it. However, I have increasingly learned to go my own way and get satisfaction from events others might regard as incredibly trivial or mundane – going for a walk with Jack or his delight the day he mastered scribbling.
> *Ruth*

Research shows that undue stress doesn't have to be part of bringing up a child with Down's syndrome, although it is true that extra problems do cause stress, such as medical problems or lack of money or support. As regards any other children, having a brother or sister with Down's syndrome seems largely to be associated with positive factors. There is no evidence that brothers and sisters develop more behavioural problems than in other families – in fact, on the whole, research indicates that they accept their different sibling as a part of the family and may be more considerate for it.

Down's syndrome and the family

Having a child with Down's syndrome by no means has to affect the family negatively. Indeed, in one of the largest, most detailed studies of Down's syndrome ever, families came out very well, undergoing much the same pressures and life situations as other families, and not finding that there was a huge difference just because of Down's syndrome. 'The overriding impression is one of normality', says the study's author, Cliff Cunningham, Visiting Professor of Applied Psychology at Liverpool John Moores University. This is not to belittle the difficulties families may face, but, rather, pay tribute to their commitment to their children.

The work of Professor Cunningham and his colleagues with the Manchester Down Syndrome Cohort began in 1973 and has continued into the children's early adulthood. It was assumed that families would automatically suffer if a child had a disability, but this was not found to be the case, in spite of children having a wide range of individual differences in terms of their mental, social and physical abilities, as well as their health and personality. 'The evidence,' concludes Professor Cunningham, 'points to positive effects where one member of the family has Down syndrome.'

The majority of families – up to 70 per cent – were tightly knit and content, with relatively normal levels of stress. They had adapted positively to having a child with Down's syndrome and were likely to feel that the child had contributed a great deal to the family. Difficulties were more likely if other aspects of life were negative, such as poor family relationships, financial strains, friction between parents, work problems, depression or illness in the parents.

Professor Cunningham identified various forms of intervention that should be put in place as early as possible to help not just those with Down's syndrome but their families as a whole. Intervention should cover a wide range of family needs, from supportive counselling to respite care, and professional help with development and behaviour management.

Research has suggested that, although living with a Down's syndrome sibling can be stressful at times and the other children may be involved with more care-giving activities, siblings tend to be more mature and tolerant than those who do not have a disabled child in the family. A study at the University of Queensland,

Australia, found that siblings of children with Down's syndrome tended to be kinder and have more empathy than other children.

Finally, if a baby is severely affected by Down's syndrome or has other health problems, such as heart disease or epilepsy, the overall strain on the family will be increased. Mostly, however, research suggests that the majority of children are affectionate towards their sibling with Down's syndrome while still being able to enjoy a life of their own.

Other children – what you can do to help them

There are several actions that you as parents can take to help family life run more smoothly:

- how parents feel and react is the biggest factor in how other siblings behave towards their Down's syndrome sibling, so, the more positive you are, the more positive your child will be
- open discussion helps greatly – keep other children informed, help them to cope with any negative reactions from friends or ignorance from other people generally
- involve your other children in plans, decisions and care
- make time for your other children
- meet the social and educational needs of your other children
- reassure your children in an age-related way – explaining genetics and reassuring them that they have not caused the condition
- other children may also occasionally appreciate time spent alone with you, without the child who has Down's syndrome.

Ways in which to reduce stress

There are many ways in which you can reduce stress, most of which mean taking time for yourself, even if it's just a few minutes. They include exercise, meditation and prayer, breathing and relaxation exercises, keeping a diary, spending time alone with your partner and so on.

Friends are key here:

Time and again, friends have saved my life and kept me going, whether it's a chat on the phone, a cup of coffee or taking the baby for an hour. Some friends have become part of the family. You do have to sort the wheat from the chaff! Unfortunately, not everyone can handle a child with special needs and, fair enough,

it's not for everyone, but for those who've stuck around, they're gold dust and I'd also say that they've found it very rewarding and warming, too.
Moira

If you are feeling overwhelmed by the demands of your child and other difficulties, counselling is an option to consider. Just talking to someone can really help you to clarify areas of confusion and set priorities.

Finally, get help – any help going, from social services, support groups or other agencies. Even if it takes the last ounce of energy you have left and you are exasperated by waiting lists, paperwork and bureaucracy, it is worth it in the long run (for more on this, see under Getting help, below). Remember, too, that support groups can help with advice and/or emotional support.

Here are some other stress busters:

- ensure that any intervention required is put in place as early as possible – it's been said before, but is worth repeating, consult your family doctor, health visitor or other relevant professional
- plan for your child's future – a significant source of stress for parents is anxiety about their child's future, so do what you can now (see under Planning your child's long-term care, below)
- planning your finances can also relieve anxiety.

Getting help

Get all the help you can and take advantage of any offers of support or babysitting. Breaks are vital as they help you to recharge your batteries and gain the strength needed to deal with the many demands of daily life.

Support groups
Seeking out local support groups and learning as much as you can about Down's syndrome can be major sources of strength.

In the UK, the Down's Syndrome Association has already been mentioned as being an excellent support group and it has a very wide range of information and support for people with Down's syndrome and their families. This and other support groups can give detailed advice on rights and benefits and how to access them.

Respite and residential care

As many people with Down's syndrome now grow up to lead independent or semi-independent lives, some parents find it wise to plan times when their child can practice living away from them for a short while. As well as giving them a stimulating change of scene, planned time apart can help families to rest and re-energize. No matter how dearly you love your child, there's no denying that a short break is sometimes needed!

Time away can be arranged in various ways – perhaps with the help of relatives or close friends who may enjoy having your child to stay for a while or else specially organized holidays for children with special needs. What is available varies from region to region, but two good starting points for information are the Down's Syndrome Association and the Family Fund (see the Useful addresses section at the back of the book for contact details).

If you want to consider more formal respite care – perhaps if your child has other difficulties and is very demanding – it is a good idea to contact your local social services for information. Do this sooner rather than later as this type of care tends to be in short supply in the UK. A support group such as the DSA may also be able to provide helpful details about how to access respite care.

Some parents feel guilty when considering whether or not to let their child go for a short break. However, you shouldn't do – as well as giving you a break, there is growing recognition that it is good for your child, too, both in the short and the long term. As well as bolstering their confidence and independence now, time away from you also means that, if a crisis does arise in the future, your child will know better how to cope. It can also pave the way for their future life, whether that's total independence, some form of sheltered housing or other residential care.

Family care

Some parents who dislike the idea of putting their child into care may, consciously or unconsciously, be relying on other family members to help or to take over as care givers. You do need to be very sure that this is indeed what they want. While it is important to involve others, such as grandparents and other children, in decisions and plans for your child with Down's syndrome, it is vital that no one feels duty-bound to take over the child's care at some future point.

Parents know that they provide their child with exceptional care and fear that no one will take care of their child in the same way if they become ill or too old to do the job. A difficult task to bequeath at the best of times, it is one that may be beyond other family members, too.

It is important to get these concerns out into the open and make a plan. Some parents form a contract with a professional guardian, who agrees to look after the interests of the person with Down's syndrome, such as observing birthdays and arranging for care.

Other sources of help

In the UK, the social services may be able to provide a range of other forms of help, such as community care, a plan that considers various needs, such as accommodation, healthcare, education, home help, help with travel and holidays, funding and grants. What the social services don't provide is treatment. See the Useful addresses section at the back of the book for contact details.

In the UK, you may be able to claim welfare benefits depending on individual circumstances. The main benefits include the Carer's Allowance, whereby councils can set up payments for parents or guardians of a disabled child (visit www.carers.gov.uk for more information), and the Disability Living Allowance (DLA), which may be claimed for a child with a severe physical or mental illness or disability if they need much more help or looking after than other children of the same age because of these issues. You also need to find out about the extra money you are entitled to for having a disabled child, in the form of the Child Tax Credit (visit the Inland Revenue site at www.taxcredits.inlandrevenue.gov.uk – you can even apply for it online). Also, contact the Department for Work and Pensions (DWP) – formerly the Department for Social Security, the DSS. Its website includes advice for those bringing up a child with special needs (visit www.dwp.gov.uk) and forms to download. Otherwise, contact your local DWP office or Post Office or Citizens Advice Bureau or ring the Benefit Enquiry Line (0800 882200).

Most applicants do eventually receive the Disability Living Allowance, says the DSA, and its welfare benefits advisers can help if you are having a problem with your claim. Disability Living Allowance can be claimed from the age of 3 months and may need to be made then if your child has a medical problem; otherwise, probably most claims should be made when your child is between 6 and 12 months old. If you are refused DLA, there is action you can take. Contact the DSA and/or look at its guidelines to claiming DLA at its website (see the Useful addresses section at the back of the book for the address).

Some charitable organizations give financial help to families with a disabled child, though, unfortunately, they cannot meet all demands. One is the Family Fund (see the Useful addresses section at the back of the book for contact details) or get in touch with the DSA, whose advisers use a computer database to find grant-making organizations suitable for your situation.

Planning your child's long-term care

Many people with Down's syndrome grow up to lead full, happy lives with a large measure of independence, taking jobs and living life to the full. Realistically, however, some form of long-term care is likely to be a reality for increasing numbers of people with Down's syndrome – whether it is total care of their physical and emotional needs or a modicum required for your child to lead an independent life with dignity. Because people with Down's syndrome live so much longer than in the past, it may be relevant to plan ahead for a time when you may become too frail to care for your child yourself or make provision for your child in the event of your death.

As individuals with Down's syndrome vary so much in their abilities and personalities, only you can judge what kind of future planning may be relevant. Most parents, however, will at some point wish to provide for their children – indeed, all their children – in the event of their illness or death. Understandably, you may shrink from the thought of planning any future, especially if your child is fragile, perhaps suffering from heart disease or other health complication, but it is best not to leave things to chance.

The following steps are suggestions that may help you to start to organize your thoughts. If possible, ask someone to help you, such as family or friends, your doctor or child's other carers or seek professional help via governmental agencies, organizations or local support groups.

- Draft out a life plan. With family and friends, decide what you want for your child in terms of residential needs, employment, education, social activities and medical care.
- Write it down. Include information about, and contact numbers for, doctors, dentists, medicine, how able your child is to function normally, types of activities enjoyed, daily living skills and rights and values.
- Write down short, clear notes or make a video of everyday activities, such as bathing, dressing, feeding, toileting, play and how your child communicates.
- Consider legal issues, such as provision for the child in your will, trustees, guardians and who will manage money matters and benefits for your child, as well as care costs and other decisions.
- Work out the cost. Calculate your monthly expenses, then work out how much will be needed to provide enough funds to support your child's lifestyle. Don't forget to include disability income, other benefits and so on.
- Research what resources are available to help you. Possibilities include government benefits, family assistance, inheritances, savings, life insurance and investments.
- Prepare legal documents. Choose a qualified lawyer to help you prepare wills, trusts, power of attorney, guardianship and so on.
- Give copies of the relevant documents and instructions to family and those involved in your child's care.
- Review your plan regularly – at least once a year. Look through and update the plan and modify legal documents as necessary.

Even if you do not do all of the above, making a will with clear provision for your child can only give you more peace of mind – perhaps the more important as, in the UK, one person in two dies without having made a will. If you prefer, another possible way to make a will is by using a will pack, which will contain background information on the law relating to intestacy (dying without having made a will), as well as important issues to consider, such as appointing an executor, specific gifts and legacies, and tax considerations. If you wish to learn more about the will-making procedure, visit www.thewillsite.co.uk for a wide range of information on the subject.

Some final thoughts

Before having Freddie, I had little perception of Down's syndrome beyond a vague idea of grim outings with children in duffle coats shuffling along. But, at a very deep level, Freddie is just another child. I realized this clearly one day when, despite Freddie's limited speech, he and his brother were having a raging argument about who should get the freebie in the cereal packet.
Annabel

As Professor Cliff Cunningham has pointed out in his major study with the Manchester Down Syndrome Cohort, families face very real problems after the birth of a child with Down's syndrome: trauma after the birth, followed by a process of massive adaptation to a new role as parents of a child with a major disability. They often face a society that barely understands Down's syndrome. They may need to learn new skills in order to deal with professionals and obtain the best resources for their child.

On an ongoing basis, they also have to stay positive and hopeful and be creative in solving problems in the face of set-backs, discouragement and slow progress. In this study, the majority of the families – who were very diverse – emerged as transcendently normal. They were subject to the same factors influencing well-being as any family and largely positive about their child. 'The fact that so many families cope well is a testimony to their commitment to their child, and their adaptability and strengths, rather than a lack of problems', says Professor Cunningham.

The study raises interesting questions about personal and cultural flexibility with regard to coping with disability. It is often said that children with Down's syndrome today have a far greater potential for learning and making a contribution to society than was believed to be possible even 10 to 15 years ago. This is fine, so long as it is not intended to have redemptive value – that is, those with Down's syndrome are now somehow deemed more acceptable because they can function in society rather than being a burden on it or that they are in danger of only being valued according to their social usefulness. This point is poignantly underlined by the conclusions of a piece of research.

In early 2003, two American professors from the University of Medicine and Dentistry of New Jersey published a study in the *New England Journal of Medicine* that identified a Flemish painting of 1515 as being possibly one of the earliest portrayals of Down's syndrome. 'The Adoration of the Christ Child' features an angel, a shepherd and possibly a cherub that seem to show features of the syndrome, such as a flattish face, eyes with epicanthic folds, a small nose and short fingers. The painting, by a follower of Jan Joest of Kalkar, is in New York's Metropolitan Museum of Art. The study's authors, Andrew Levitas and Cheryl Reid, speculate as to whether or not those with Down's syndrome in the sixteenth century were even recognized as having what we now call intellectual disability, if they were treated differently by society or if the whole issue was not relevant. People with mild forms of the syndrome might merely have been perceived as being slightly slow and might have been fully integrated into society, suggest the authors: 'He or she, or they, could well have been beloved or at least accepted in a family or village group, even a member of the unknown artist's family.' They conclude, 'After all the speculations, we are left with a haunting late-medieval image of a person with apparent Down syndrome with all the accoutrements of divinity.'

Further reading

Beck, Martha (2000) *Expecting Adam: A True Story of Birth, Rebirth, and Everyday Magic*. New York: Berkley Publishing Group.

Bérubé, M. (1998) *Life as We Know It: A Father, a Family and an Exceptional Child*. New York: Vintage Books.

Bruni, M. (1998) *Fine Motor Skills in Children with Down Syndrome: A guide for Parents and Professionals*. Bethesda, Maryland: Woodbine House.

Buckley, Sue (1986) *The Development of Language and Reading Skills in Children with Down's Syndrome*. Portsmouth: The Sarah Duffen Centre, Portsmouth Polytechnic.

Byrne, Elizabeth A., Cunningham, Cliff C., and Sloper, Patricia (1988) *Families and their Children with Down's Syndrome: One Feature in Common*. New York: Routledge.

Carr, Janet (1995) *Down's Syndrome: Children Growing Up*. Cambridge: Cambridge University Press.

Cunningham, Cliff C. (1996) *Understanding Down Syndrome: An Introduction for Parents*. Cambridge, Massachusetts: Brookline Books.

Dyke, Don C. Van (1995) *Medical and Surgical Care for Children with Down Syndrome: A Guide for Parents*. Bethesda, Maryland: Woodbine House.

Fujita, H. (1990) *Fitness Exercises for the Down's Syndrome Baby*. Osaka, Japan: Jordan Co.

Kingsley, Jason, and Levitz, Mitchell (1994) *Count Us In: Growing up with Down Syndrome*. Orlando, Florida: Harcourt Publishers.

Kumin, Libby (1994) *Communication Skills in Children with Down Syndrome: A Guide for Parents*. Bethesda, Maryland: Woodbine House.

Kumin, Libby (2001) *Classroom Language Skills for Children with Down Syndrome: A Guide for Parents and Teachers*. Bethesda, Maryland: Woodbine House.

Lejeune, Clara (2001) *Life is a Blessing: A Biography of Jérôme Lejeune – Geneticist, Doctor, Father*. Fort Collins, Colorado: Ignatius Press.

Marino, B., and Pueschel, S. M. (eds) (1996) *Heart Disease in Persons with Down Syndrome*. Baltimore, Maryland: Paul H. Brookes Publishing Co.

Medlen, Joan E. Guthrie (2002) *The Down Syndrome Nutrition Handbook: A Guide to Promoting Healthy Lifestyles*. Bethesda, Maryland: Woodbine House.

Mepsted, Joyce (1998) *Developing the Child with Down's Syndrome: A Guide for Teachers, Parents and Carers*. Plymouth: Northcote House.

Merriman, A. (1999) *A Minor Adjustment*. London: Pan Macmillan.

Parker, James N., and Parker, Phillip M. (eds) (2002) *The 2002 Official Parent's Sourcebook on Down Syndrome*. San Diego, California: ICON Health Publications.

Pueschel, Siegfried M. (ed.) (1988) *The Young Person with Down Syndrome*. Kingston-upon-Thames: Kluwer Academic and Plenum Publishers.

Pueschel, Siegfried M. (ed.) (1991) *A Parent's Guide to Down Syndrome: Toward a Brighter Future*. Baltimore, Maryland: Paul H. Brookes Publishing Co.

Rogers, Paul, and Coleman, Mary (1992) *Medical Care in Down Syndrome: A Preventive Medicine Approach*. New York: Dekker.

Selikowitz, Mark (1997) *Down Syndrome: The Facts*. Oxford: Oxford University Press.

Stray-Gundersen, Karen (ed.) (1995) *Babies with Down Syndrome: A New Parent's Guide*. Bethesda, Maryland: Woodbine House.

Sumar, Sonia, Volk, Jeffrey, and Marusso, Adriana (1998) *Yoga for the Special Child: A Therapeutic Approach for Infants & Children with Down Syndrome, Cerebral Palsy and Learning Disabilities*. Buckingham, Virginia: Special Yoga Publications.

Ward, O. Conor (1998) *Eponymists in Medicine: John Langdon Down 1828–1896 – A Caring Pioneer*. London: Royal Society of Medicine Press.

Ward, O. Conor (1999) 'John Langdon Down (1828–1896)', in F. Clifford Rose (ed.), *A Short History of Neurology*. London: Butterworth Heinemann.

Winders, Patricia (1997) *Gross Motor Skills in Children with Down Syndrome: A Guide for Parents and Professionals*. Bethesda, Maryland: Woodbine House.

Useful addresses

Down's Syndrome Association
Langdon Down Centre
2a Langdon Park
Teddington TW11 9PS
Tel: 0845 230 0372
Fax: 0845 230 0372
Website: www.downs-syndrome.org.uk
E-mail: info@downs-syndrome.org.uk

DSA Wales
Suite 1
206 Whitechurch Road
Heath
Cardiff
South Glamorgan CF4 3NB
Tel: 029 2052 2511
Fax: 029 2052 2511
E-mail: dsa.wales@lineone.net

DSA Northern Ireland
Graham House
Knockbracken Healthcare Park
Saintfield Road
Belfast BT8 8BH
Tel: 028 9070 4606
Fax: 028 9070 4075
E-mail: downs-syndrome@cinni.org

Down Syndrome Educational Trust
Sarah Duffen Centre
Belmont Street
Southsea
Hampshire PO5 1NA
Tel: 023 9285 5330

Fax: 023 9285 5320
Website: www.downsed.org
E-mail: enquiries@downsed.org
E-mail is the preferred means of contact – visit the website for additional specific addresses.

Down's Heart Group
17 Cantilupe Close
Eaton Bray
Dunstable
Bedfordshire LU6 2EA
Tel: 01525 220379
Fax: 01525 221553
Website: www.downs-heart.downsnet.org
E-mail: downs_heart_group@msn.com

Down's Syndrome Scotland
158/160 Balgreen Road
Edinburgh EH11 3AU
Tel: 0131 313 4225
Fax: 0131 313 4285
Website: www.dsscotland.org.uk
E-mail: info@dsscotland.org.uk

Down's Clinic (formerly the Lejeune Clinic)
Hospital of St John and St Elizabeth
60 Grove End Road
London NW8 9NH
Tel: 020 7286 5126, extension 413
Fax: 020 7266 4813
Website: www.jamont.freeserve.co.uk/lejeune
E-mail: advice@lejeuneclinic.org

Association for Post Natal Illness
145 Dawes Road
Fulham
London SW6 7EB
Tel: 020 7386 0868 (helpline)
Fax: 020 7386 8885
Website: www.apni.org
E-mail: info@apni.org

Euro-TNS
Beannachar Camphill Community
South Deeside Road
Banchory Devenick
Aberdeen AB12 5YL
Tel: 01224 869251
Fax: 01224 869251
Website: www.beannachar.co.uk
E-mail: richard.beannachar.org
TNS stands for Targeted Nutritional Support (similar to TNI). The
product is sold on a cost basis with the expectation that parents will
provide financial support for medical research initiated by the DSRF.
Please consult your doctor before buying this product. The UK
mainland prices are:
£27.00 for adult size (320 g)
£8.30 for child size (100 g)
for postage and packing add £2.00, but for orders over £50, shipping
is free.

Family Fund
PO Box 50
York YO1 9ZX
Tel: 0845 130 4542
Fax: 01904 652 625
Website: www.familyfundtrust.org.uk
E-mail: info@familyfund.org.uk

Footprints Holiday House
Stodmarsh Road
Canterbury
Kent CT3 4AP
Tel: 01227 780796 or 785067
Fax: 01227 764480
Website: www.miles-of-smiles.org.uk
E-mail: admin@footprints-holidays.org.uk

Leukaemia CARE
2 Shrubbery Avenue
Worcester WR1 1QH
Tel: 0800 169 6680 (24-hour helpline)
Fax: 01905 330090
Website: www.leukaemiacare.org
E-mail: enquiries@leukaemiaCARE.org.uk

National Childbirth Trust
Alexandra House
Oldham Terrace
Acton
London W3 6NH
Tel: 0870 444 8707 (enquiry line)
Fax: 0870 770 3237
Website: www.nct-online.org

SNAP
Keys Hall
Eagle Way
Warley
Brentwood
Essex CM13 3BP
Tel: 01277 211300
Fax: 01277 212333
Website: www.snapcharity.org
E-mail: info@snapcharity.org
Support group for parents of children with special needs and
disabilities. Visit the website for a directory of respite care.

North America

National Down Syndrome Society
666 Broadway
New York, NY 10012
Tel: 212 460 9330
Fax: 212 979 2873
Website: www.ndss.org
E-mail: info@ndss.org

National Down Syndrome Congress
1370 Center Drive
Suite 102
Atlanta, GA 30338
Tel: 800 232 NDSC or 770 604 9500
Website: www.ndsccenter.org
E-mail: info@ndsccenter.org

Down Syndrome Research Foundation
1409 Sperling Avenue
Burnaby, BC V5B 4J8
Tel: 604 444 3773 or 1 888 464 DSRF
Fax: 604 431 9248
Website: www.dsrf.org
E-mail: info@dsrf.org

Downi Creations, Inc.
410 Steeple Crest North
Irmo, SC 29063
Tel: 1 888 749 9330 or 803 749 9330
Fax: 803 749 2752
Website: www.downicreations.com
E-mail: DOWNI96@aol.com
Makers of Down's syndrome dolls.

Europe

Jérôme Lejeune Foundation
Fondation Jérôme Lejeune
31 rue Galande
75005 Paris
France
Tel: 01 46 33 31 82
Website: www.fondationlejeune.org
E-mail: fjl@fondationlejeune.org

Other useful websites

Alzheimer's Society
Website: www.alzheimers.org.uk

Autism Independent UK
Website: www.autismuk.com

British Deaf Association
Website: www.britishdeafassociation.org.uk

British Thyroid Foundation
Website: www.btf-thyroid.org

Diabetes support groups
Website: www.diabetes.org.uk

Down's Syndrome Medical Interest Group (DSMIG)
Website: www.dsmig.org.uk

Down Syndrome WWW page
Website: www.nas.com/downsyn/start.html

Miriam Kauk's comprehensive and useful website
Website: www.einstein-syndrome.com

International Rare Disease Support Network
Website: www.raredisorders.com

Hirschsprungs & Motility Disorders Support Network, The Guardian Society
Website: www.theguardiansociety.org
Hirschsprung's disease support groups.

La Lèche League
Website: www.lalecheleague.org
For the booklet 'Breastfeeding the Baby with Down Syndrome'.

International Mosaic Down Syndrome Association
Website: www.imdsa.com

National Society for Epilepsy
Website: www.epilepsynse.org.uk

Riverbend Down Syndrome Parent Support Group
Website: www.altonweb.com/cs/downsyndrome
Timeline:
www.altonweb.com/cs/downsyndrome/timeline.html

Genetics Education Center at the University of Kansas Medical Center
Website: www.kumc.edu/gec/support/down-syn.html
International and very extensive source of contacts and links.

Living with Reflux
Website: http://groups.msn.com/LivingWithRefluxUK
Reflux support group.

Sleep Apnoea Trust
Website: www.sleep-apnoea-trust.org

Young Down's Group
Website: www.paston.co.uk/users/maygurney/dsa.html

Trisomy 21 Online Community
Website: http://trisomy21online.com

Index